Fitface

Hands Free
Facial Toning Exercises

Charlotte Hamilton

Published in the United Kingdom
By
Fitface

For bulk order purchases or for other information please visit
www.fitfacetoning.com

Typeset, printed and bound in the United Kingdom

By the same author under the pseudonym

Colette Sinclair

MAN HUNT

First published: Sidgwick and Jackson - Pan Macmillan Press 1989

This book is a work of non-fiction and a true story.

To respect the sensibilities of some people and the professional careers of others I have elected to purposefully withhold some names throughout the book.

Liability Waiver

Fitface Toning Inc accepts no responsibility or liability for any injury, loss or damage to any party undertaking or performing the facial exercises, stretches or procedures set out within this book and all parties undertake and perform such exercises, movements, stretches and procedures entirely at their own risk.

The reader further acknowledges, agrees and understands that the information here within is for reference and education only and not in any way intended to be a substitute for a physician's advice, diagnosis or treatment.

For my daughter Brittany whom I love madly

and

Nami wherever he may be.

With special thanks to:

Captain Peter: he listened and encouraged me to finish.
Coco: she inspired me to continue to tell the world,
"There is another way to look beautiful forever."
Mummie and Brian Blunden: for editing.
They all made this book possible.

About the Author

Born and raised in England. Charlotte immigrated to California USA in her twenties. There she witnessed firsthand the butchery of a major face-lift to her former partner and vowed never to have a face-lift. Following the breakup of her marriage she returned to England to raise her new baby daughter. Eighteen years later, her daughter suffered a horrendous near fatal accident in which she sustained major facial trauma with 21 fractures to her face. She survived, graduated with an honours' degree and now lives in Australia. Charlotte returned to live in Florida, USA.

Charlotte loves to hear from readers and will endeavour to answer every single e-mail. She invites you to visit her website at **www.Fitfacetoning.com**

Hands Free
Facial Toning Exercises

Foreword

Fitface - The natural face-lift, a guide to hands free facial toning exercises is not just a "How to" book. It is in part a very personal autobiographical story, told to you in such a way as to be real, heartfelt and not edited by some professional writer; it comes from the heart, my heart, me, Charlotte Hamilton. They are my words, my feelings and thoughts. Hopefully, you will identify with some parts here within and therefore be encouraged to not only start the facial toning exercises but also to continue with a maintenance programme, the results of which will make you an advocate of facial exercises for life.

Contents

Part 1

Why do Fitface?

Information you should know

Chapter 5

Facial Surgery and Alternatives

Part 2

FACE EXERCISES

With photographs showing you how to exercise

Chapter 6

The Foundations

Chapter 7

Basic Fitface exercise training programme   143

Chapter 8

Step 1 Anytime Fitface toning programme   157

Chapter 9

Chapter 10

Chapter 11

Information

Part 1

Why do Fitface?

Information you should know

Chapter 1

The Beginning

Witnessing a face-lift with eyelid surgery

Back in the late seventies face-lifts and boob jobs were the latest fad, or so we thought then, in California, which was where I was living as a resident although originally born and raised in England. At that time not much was known about cosmetic surgery except that surgery could make you look like an entirely different person. The "stars", as they were then called, were having face-lifts done, and they were publicised as relatively pain free and very, very, expensive, therefore making them the latest "must have" for the young, rich, totally impressionable, courageous, brave beyond reason, irresponsible and pitifully unknowingly, beautiful things of my generation. More to the point face-lifts and boob jobs were essential for those us of us within the "in-crowd" who were not so very beautiful, which superbly fitted the description of my ex boyfriend Nami in every way.

My boyfriend was from Saudi Arabia; educated, intelligent, wealthy and self indulgent. He was always festooned in the finest of European tailoring despite his small frame and although he could be adorably kind, however only to me, was one of the most hideous men on the planet. Not only was he plain ugly but he had seriously droopy, folded jowls on the side of his face, just like a "hush puppy dog" considered cute on them but the same would not be an adjective one could readily describe him with hideous? Yes. He knew it, and he called himself the "runt of the litter," having explained that his mother had had 19 other children and he drew the short straw! Our break up was to come 2 years later after I had met the most handsome, gorgeous, sexiest man on the planet, a Latino hunk named Raymond, who seemed only to have ever worn jeans and a Stetson. Me, being young and fat thinking I was IN LOVE, rather than lust; I fled and left Nami for the arms of this unbelievable super stud.

A few months later, after I had been hiding in fear of what Nami might do, thinking perhaps he'd kill me for leaving, (his emotions were not to be trifled with) I had agreed to meet him. That was only because he had caught me - stopped at a red light on PCH (Pacific Coast Highway) and had thrown himself on the hood of my car and pleaded to be heard. Unbeknown to me, he had concocted in his head, the idea that if he was to win me back he had better look like Raymond and had elected to have cosmetic surgery. He told me all about what the surgeons had said and I was actually all for it. It sounded great, simple and easy. I naively thought that if he got rid of the jowls he would look better and therefore attract more women, meet someone else and get over me. I am now older and wiser and hopefully can forgive myself for being as naïve as that in my mid twenties. He had oodles of money and if it made him look better why not?

The day of the surgery he had begged me to pick him up. How could I refuse? I thought it was the least I could do I may have even said the same to Raymond. At the appointed time, I arrived at the sumptuous, austere offices of Orange County's most eminent plastic surgeon housed in the prestigious medical centre and was plied with refreshments whilst I waited. I was informed it had taken longer than anticipated and that Nami had been difficult. Nothing new there, I thought. The door opened and there sat Nami pathetically in a wheelchair with a head the size of a pumpkin, all bound up in layer upon layer of brown crepe bandages; I was stunned. He looked wretched, worse still; he was trying to call my name, mumbling "Charlotte… Charlotte," through the vague split in his bandages where his mouth was, weakly extending a flaying arm in the air tragically searching for me.

"He has been extremely difficult" the surgeon said curtly. Muttering something about taking 2 inches of skin from each side and it had been radical surgery. Nami meantime, drugged up, which was not his style, was desperately trying to pull at his bandages and get out of his wheelchair. Unlike my normal behaviour, I quickly sought his hand and held it tightly while reassuring him I was there. The site of him hard torn at my heartstrings, I felt so guilty, not that it was my idea in the first place, but that I had encouraged him and secretly thought that if he looked good when it was over, then maybe I could have my eyes done. I had always fancied larger eyes. It had all seemed so simple when he first told me.

Muffled by the bandages, I could only barely make out Nami weeping with delight and gratitude at having found me there. I felt even worse, he looked so pathetic. In my defence, we had been separated for months and besides, I was living with another man! He was excited, desperately trying to talk through the opening made for his mouth in the bandages. He was

2

so eager for me to see the results. Hurriedly, he continued to pull at the separate pile of bandages that were the foremost, covering his eyes just to see me. Seeing his distress I helped him unwind what I thought was that portion. As we did so, the white inner cotton gauze pads that were covering his eyes fell away, covered in blood, I saw the stitches below his swollen weeping eyes where they had pulled up his lower eye lid bags I felt sickened, my knees weakened and I fell faint into an easy chair.

When I had recovered, I called a friend of ours to collect both of us. We took Nami home and I hired a nurse to look after him as there was no way that I could put his eye drops in. I couldn't even look at him without feeling nauseous despite only his eyes and lips showing. Most of the bandages were still on. I could not act as his nurse. I was so utterly ashamed of myself and yet it was he that was in pain!

Days later, when all the bandages came off he looked horrific and I will never forget the state of his face. Dried blood, huge scars, swelling, lumpy stitches and bruising – they were not a pretty sight and that was not the result he had expected. His nurse was wonderful, changing his dressings, giving him his medications, and sponge bathing him. He had discovered some relief from his oh so stretched skin by applying a face cloth soaked in tepid water that enabled him to move his whole face again. Slowly he recovered as the days ran into weeks and as the weeks turned into months he gradually healed.

The eventual outcome was that, where once he had an animated expression, fuelled by emotion and a vibrant face, there was none, just a taut mask. Where before there had been a head full of thick dark brown hair, there was none, it had been replaced by a Pope's cap size clump of hair on top of the rear of his head. His normal hairline had been pulled back and up, so far, in every direction, that his beard was now to grow behind his ears! He was mutilated, which is exactly what a face-lift is... self mutilation and for what? Feeling good for a few years? From then on, I consciously vowed never to have a face-lift.

As the months passed he healed further, he grew his hair to cover the baldness and I got used to the sight of him and within a year hardly even noticed his disfigurement. However, it was Nami who had to live with the consequences and although the constant feeling of tightness caused by his taut skin did eventually subside and finally disappeared, sadly that was not so with the initial numbness he felt down one side of his face. He

3

thought that would ease with the passing months and be completely alleviated, it did, to some extent. But for the first couple of years, he had to be especially careful about what and how he ate. If he wasn't careful he would unintentionally take chunks out of the side of his cheeks whenever he chewed voraciously. However, the twinges and nerve damage that he had experienced at first, although they had improved over time, had never really ceased, even 20 years later, which was the last time I saw him.

I can fully appreciate that in the last 30 years there have been significant improvements in all areas of medical science, not just cosmetic surgery. However, I was obviously "put off" for life about the consequences of having a face-lift or eyelid surgery after that experience. Although I was not responsible for Nami's decision to have a face-lift, to this day I still feel a shadow of guilt that someone loved me enough to intentionally allow themselves to be put through all that pain to try to please me.

Whenever my old mother and I watched TV together and a programme about facial surgery came up she always said, "Don't you ever have anything like that done, if you do I'll never speak to you again!" It's funny but it's one of the few times that I don't jump down her throat for trying to be dictatorial or controlling, instead I strangely feel loved. If I loved someone, I would not want to see them to go through unnecessary cosmetic surgery and would not support their decision without voicing my strong objections. Surely I would love them as themselves, for what they are. I do find it extremely difficult to comprehend the opposite opinion when I hear people encourage their friends, lovers, spouses or family to have surgery. Can that truly be love?

Creating Fitface toning

When and how I started hands free facial exercises

A few years passed and I was still living in California. In the early eighties the aerobic exercise craze was in full swing and like everyone else I was into strenuously working out from the neck down. I practised all the latest exercise routines until I knew them by heart. I was obsessed with being slim and looking great, which made me feel that I belonged to the "In" crowd. The media coverage of what celebrities looked like wasn't as intense as it is today but I still felt compelled to compete with these unknown airbrushed photographic beauties. I was terrified of getting old and ugly and being forced to have a face-lift, I just couldn't do it, not with the barbarity of Nami's ordeal so freshly impinged on my memory. Therefore I looked into all alternative methods to stay youthful looking. There was and is no way I could go through what he went through. Far too scary and I am not good with pain.

At that time, quite by chance I came across a book of facial exercises written by a doctor. I believe it was called something like The15 minute face-lift. It seemed to make perfect sense to me. I began to try out the exercises but I couldn't be bothered to keep them up and put the book away. I preferred to use expensive creams, and fast tanning oils on the beach or at the sun tanning salon. Despite living in California sun beds were all the rage, I even owned them in a hair salon so I was on them constantly. I kept my weight down with an addiction to Diet sodas, diet foods and diet pills none of which are exactly ideal nutrition for the skin!

By the mid Eighties I was pregnant. Gave birth to a beautiful baby girl and returned home to England, to live with my mother.

Fortunately, I had taken the facial exercise book with me. By the age of 34 I was beginning to become increasingly concerned about the emergence of unsightly frown lines, furrows on my forehead and folds from my nose to my chin that were beginning to appear on my face. In desperation, I sought out my old book and returned to doing what was then considered my silly facial exercises and amazingly the wrinkles seemed to disappear!

I told all my friends who initially thought, as secretly did I, that this was yet another fad for me to get obsessed with and then forget. But it wasn't, I became engrossed and began practicing facial exercises every day. I bought a video, other facial exercise books and experimented with a whole array of techniques gradually becoming more and more competent. In time, I became totally proficient and had taught myself which exercises worked the best and which ones did nothing at all.

Back then when I did my facial exercises even my mother would say "You'll stretch your skin and regret it" but now under duress she will reluctantly admit, especially since the resurgent of interest in preventative measures to the knife, that there may be something in it and on occasion even goes so far as to condone them!. Unforgiving, I remind her constantly about facial exercises whenever she makes comments about how old some people look that are considerably younger than me.

In the early days my girlfriends just laughed at me and made jokes, pulling contorted faces but now 20 years later it is I who have the last laugh, as I do indeed look younger than they do - please excuse me - to all those whom I refer. You know who you are and what I mean, hopefully you will forgive me.

It will soon be twenty years since I began my quest to find an alternative to the knife. Some of my friends, who still haven't taken my advice and started exercising, would like to believe that it's all in the genes, perhaps so. I'll never know. My mother use to hold on to the gene theory but not anymore, finally she is convinced. She is a large woman and now elderly and as such she has a very large neck and jowls, so the theory is difficult to prove. All I know for certain is that when I stop doing facial exercises, even for a little while, due to work commitments or holidays, I begin to notice that my face looks just a little more tired and less toned, so I don't stop but start again. I am 100% certain they work.

Over the years I have researched numerous different books, videos, talked to surgeons all over the world, and experiment with various different methods of facial exercise. Some facial exercises I liked more than others, some, I thought were more useful than others and occasionally I found ones that were either too difficult to master or were too complicated to remember. Eventually, I settled on an assortment of the exercises that I found to be the most effective and produced different basic routines to keep my interest level high. They must be enjoyable and fun in order to stick with them.

Gradually I began to tell more and more people about doing my facial exercises and how great they were. A few listened, most did not, in the early days most people thought that I was a bit crazy but as my friends aged they showed more and more interest as my ageing seemed to be at a slower pace than theirs. Eventually, some of them responded to my offer to teach them the toning exercises and were delighted with the results. Ultimately, encouraged by their success, I decided to write a guide containing the best combination of exercises for maintaining a naturally youthful look. I wanted the book to be more personal than just a "how to exercise the face to look good" in order that you, the reader would be encouraged to keep up a maintenance programme forever. Today, I am sharing that knowledge with you in Fitface the guide to facial toning.

My final word is that for someone who has lived life right on the edge, in the sunshine state of California in her twenties (even owning a sun bed there), has spent many months in other countries such as the Bahamas and Bahrain lapping up the sun to acquire an almost dark rich tan, tried to chain smoke myself to death for over 40 years - assisted by copious amounts of alcohol/diet sodas, none of which I recommend, my face and absence of wrinkles is almost miraculous. Therefore my only logical conclusion would be to put it down to the years I've spent doing facial exercises. Logically what else could it possibly be?

The next chapter entitled the lifestyle of the author explains in far greater detail my struggles with all addictions to smoking, diet cola, food and alcohol all of which are not indicative of a lustrous wrinkle and fold free face. I have included that chapter to avert critics who may say ah yes but look at her perfect lifestyle. Yes, perhaps now I have learnt with age to be better at taking care of myself but it wasn't always the case. So if you are not at the whole food market, eating organic produce and working out everyday do not be discouraged, it's never too late to change towards a healthier lifestyle.

Lifestyle of the author

Born in 1956

Superficially I appear to be a reasonably well preserved, young looking mature woman. Someone who has never had a weight problem, with no worries and just looks that way she does because of her genes, nothing could be further from the truth. One would only have to view my upper thighs and underarms to see that I speak the truth. However this is not an autobiography. Even so I feel it is important for you to understand that I have lived life to the full and subsequently mentally endured more stress than any one person should have to and physically I have abused my body with excessive smoking and drinking for most of my life. Something I am not proud of but nonetheless remains the truth.

My first real memories of a weight problem were at about aged eight. I distinctly remember walking a few paces behind my mother who was rather beautiful but somewhat ashamed of having a fat kid in tow. My "puppy fat" was the result of too many trips to the tuck box whilst desperately unhappy at my British boarding school. I was very fat and therefore teased or rather bullied at school which of course, only made me eat more to ease my pain.

By the age of 10 it was time for me to be fitted for my new convent school uniform. I remember to this day the shame I felt as I watched my mother being forced to buy a size 16 for me, only available in the senior style dress, which would have made me stick out like a sore thumb. Fortunately she had a considerable talent as a seamstress and reluctantly she was able to stitch in extra diamonds of a similar fabric under the arms, (to accommodate my fat arms), take out the gathers of the waistband and hitch up the hem (which was almost to the floor) which at least made me look half way decent. Unfortunately that didn't deter me from buying sweets (candies) after school from the local shop.

It was at around that time, aged 10 or 11 that I first started smoking; taking the odd "drag" off of a Number 6 (cigarettes sold in packets of 10's) down to the woods with my friends, the village children. We all did, we thought we were cool and slowly from the odd "drag", to the odd pack developed into a full flung habit.

At about 14, something clicked about my weight, or perhaps, looking back I think it was to impress a young doctor who took an interest in me whom I had a crush on (or fancied). He suggested that I be put me on a grapefruit diet. Amazingly the ugly duckling became a swan and I revealed in the attention. I had lost 40lbs. I was hardly svelte, just pleasingly plump with big boobs and big bottom therefore the arduous attentions of both boys and men were not in short supply. It was then that I started going to the local country pub with my friends and my love of booze started. I felt loved, confident and invincible.

By the age of 22 I was now living in California with an Arab (who I eventually married and subsequently had that marriage annulled) and was as fat as butter; guzzling on a gallon of wine a day, smoking 40 cigarettes, not working, just lolling about, being lazy, (bone idol if truth be told) sunbathing/sun bedding in the afternoon and clubbing at night until the wee hours: a truly sophisticated party animal! All the weight had gone back on and more besides, although I had every material possession I could possibly want I was obviously very unhappy. I reached my maximum weight at 23 which was when I fell completely and utterly head over heels in love, all 182 lbs of me!

He was a beach bum who only cared about his body, a gloriously gorgeous Mexican American. Even now I can remember exactly the moment I decided to do something about my weight problem or should I say **he** decided to do something about it for me. It was in California, we had just made love and I was puffing and sweating like a whale. I looked down on my sagging flab, I was so humiliated, tears rolled down my face, I was so ashamed I just sobbed. His attitude was not one of sympathy but one of "Well let's do something about it!"

From that day on he was on a mission. That night he ran me around the block and I can remember my body's horrific, shock reaction, my heart was pounding, my skin was on fire red with the circulation, I sweated like a pig, my legs felt like jelly, I was nauseous and hated him for putting me through this which after all was only a mild jog around the block! So began my rigid exercise routine, until eventually through grit determination (and sexual obsession for my trainer) I caught the bug.

Diet wise for the next six months he starved me, even in restaurants he would order for me by saying "Oh, she will have salad" and a glass of sparkling mineral water!" Obviously I lost tons of weight, well 70 lbs and ended up a svelte size 4. Then as these things do I evened out at 120 lbs and in my mid thirties was 130 lbs which is where I remain today (but only by "watching it"). Okay maybe 134lbs.

My boyfriend openly smoked weed and secretly did cocaine (hence the energy) and therefore he complained little about my drinking, besides I had cut back somewhat. He smoked about 4 cigarettes a day so nothing was said about my smoking, which behind his back was becoming a real problem.

However, I traded my obsession with food into an unhealthy addiction to diet cola which yes I truly believe that I have paid for in cellulite and was it any wonder? As at one point I was competing with the well reported consumption of a very famous heiress drinking a minimum of a 6 pack a day. The only other long term consequence of this action was the cost of dental care. Already then known as a "bitter, slider, grinder", brace wearing patient of Guy's dental training hospital in London, my continued use only exacerbated my condition. The long term result was that now most of my teeth have been replaced with composite material because each night I wear them out; hence my visage in the mouth area is perhaps not what it should be.

At 29 I left the USA and my Mexican American partner with my month old little girl and went to live in back England to be at my mother's home. It was then that I began to become a fully fledged vegetarian. I think my long journey had begun in my childhood with a hatred of being forced to eat the gristle on red meat which had made me gag. At 18 I had stopped eating veal because while out walking with a ruggedly handsome farmer's son (on whom I was dotty), he had picked a calf (with loveable gooey eyes and a wet nose) and looking at it cradled in his arms said "Veal!" That was it; never again would I eat veal. Over the course of the next 5 years, I progressed to abstinence of eating red meat entirely and eventually to only eating white meat as it was the fashion in California.

In England I was a Mummie, working only part time. I did not feel very well generally and had arthritic pain first thing in the morning despite exercising. With more time to read about my ailments I investigated further into my aches and pains and discovered that a probable cause was diet. So I decided to experiment. I gave up eating white meat and started eating more pulses and wholemeal products. Encouraged by feeling better I no longer ate meat of any colour and was a faux vegetarian only eating fish and shell fish. As my mother did the majority of the cooking and she had always cooked "hot nutritious dinners" with 2 or more vegetables and great puddings it wasn't the hardship you might think. By the time I was about 35 I was a total vegetarian.

Living in England and being "a mother" my lifestyle had to change. The sun had gone but the northerly winds and constant use of central heating ravaged my face instead. Over the next nine years I continued working out to video tapes and took up the sport of badminton and tennis. I ate more sensibly, drank less (owing to financial restraints) but still smoked like a chimney and was still addicted to diet cola. But the excesses of the past had begun to be etched on my face. I was beginning to look old for my age. That's perhaps the reason why I started to do facial exercises in earnest at the beginning of the Nineties (aged 34) as there was no way that I would go through a face-lift after my experience with Nami.

By the mid Nineties I had met a new man, he later became my husband. We had started a business which rapidly became successful and we developed the product into an international brand leader. Hence there was constant stress and little or no time to work out and my addictions to cigarettes, booze and diet colas accelerated. The marriage was doomed to failure and upon divorce I knew I must straighten myself out.

Instantly I quit diet cola and cigarettes, although I almost became hooked on the anti smoking aid tablets! Five years later on I wouldn't dare touch a cigarette and very occasionally treat myself to a diet cola. I changed what I could; I had to as physically I was on a fast train to nowhere. The stress had eased but not abated as my husband's attitude to the acrimonious divorce was that he would bankrupt the company rather than give me a penny. At 46 I changed careers and had severe money worries paying my daughter's almost £20,000 ($40,000 – after tax) school fees (with all the extras).

However, having had climbed yet another mammoth hurdle I was only to endure a further dramatic shock and emotional trauma just a year later, when my only daughter was impaled face first on a brick wall (see later - Facial surgeries vs. facial exercise). Stress is a killer and the first visible signs are often as ageing of the skin on the face and wrinkles, I have had buckets full. But I didn't go back to smoking.

To this day I am still a vegetarian (although all nutritionists would shoot me, if they only knew what I ate, because - although I try - I fail to maintain a balanced diet). My biggest failing is that I simply can't be bothered with cooking all those pulses, mixing protein and producing a balanced diet. Luckily I pick largely on raw fruits and vegetables so there is much goodness in that alone. I figure that my body will tell me what I should eat and it usually does. Sometimes I may have a thing about pineapple, whereas another time it will be bread, it could even be cabbage and then of course there is always wine, chocolate cravings and food binges which are all too present, I am not perfect.

Booze has and always will be a problem for me. I enjoy the taste and the effects. I always have and yes, I know the risks and the damage it causes both internally and externally. What can I say? I am a middle aged, middle class drinker. In England, drinking is just part of the social norm; it's just a routine, most of my girlfriends drink ½ to a bottle of wine daily and I'm no exception. Its way too much! I'm at least trying to stop now living in the USA.

So that's it, I wasn't an angel as you will have read. My lifestyle has been somewhat excessive and just in case you were wondering, yes I am post menopausal. However despite my biological body clock age (54) and perpetual over indulgences my face doesn't show it to that extent. According to all the lifestyle magazines I should look like a haggard old lady with skin like a prune but I don't. I put this down to my constant participation in facial exercises.

My conclusion is that appearing physically attractive and healthy is all about moderation and getting balance into your life. I try to eat right - while still consuming masses of chocolate "Yummy!" and extra thick double cream with everything from bananas to brandy snaps but NOT ALL THE TIME. Fortunately in the United States I can't find any! I continued to work out sometimes more than others, be it certainly much less aerobically and much less frequently than it used to be. Now with a splattering of videos, DVD's the gym, the odd walk or swimming. Sometimes, even only accomplishing either a game of tennis or a lesson of yoga in a month! You will not find me getting up at the crack of dawn or see me after work in the gym more like the pub BUT NOT ALL THE TIME. I do try to get 7 hours of sleep a night and then have a mad couple of weeks where I am out to all hours travelling in an exciting country but NOT ALL THE TIME. I continue to do facial exercises most the time! Looking good – **is all about getting the balance right.**

Chapter 2

Face and Neck Anatomy

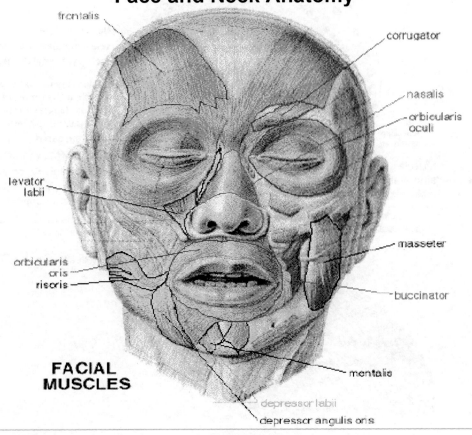

FACIAL MUSCLES

Labels on figure: frontalis, corrugator, nasalis, orbicularis oculi, levator labii, masseter, orbicularis oris, risoris, buccinator, mentalis, depressor labii, depressor angulis oris

Frontalis:	the forehead
Corrugators:	the brow
Nasalis:	the nose
Orbicularis oculi:	around the eye
Orbicularis oris:	around the mouth purses the lips
Levator labii:	raises the upper lip
Masseter:	closes the jaw
Risorius:	draws the lips in a grinning smile
Buccinator:	pulls the lips wide and tight
Depressor labii:	lowers the lower lips
Depressor anguli oris:	lowers the bottom corner of the lips
Mentalis:	pulls chin down

Image: Face and neck muscles

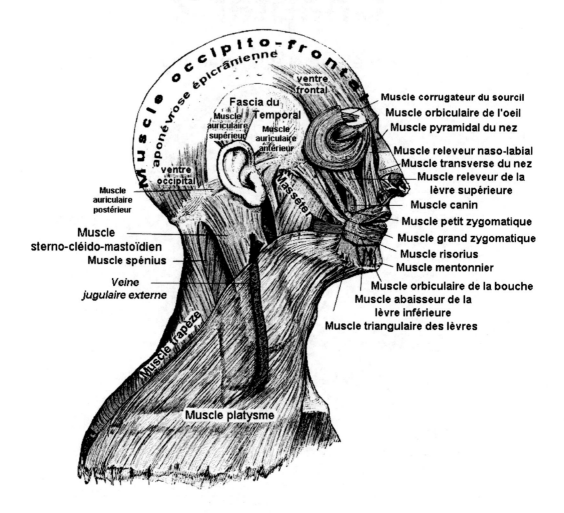

Muscle risorius
(vue latérale droite)

Risorius (side of mouth indicated above)

The *risorius* retracts the angle of the mouth to produce a smile, albeit an insincere looking one that does not involve the skin around the eyes. Compare with a genuine smile, which raises the lips with the action of zygomaticus major *and* zygomaticus minor *muscles* around the eyes using the orbicularis oculi *muscles.* This shows crow's feet when you show a real smile. The *platysma muscle* covers the front of the neck.

Muscles of the face and their actions

The **facial bones** are the foundation upon which our appearance is built, with the overlying **skin** and **muscles** adding the finishing touches, allowing us to recognise each other. Our facial expression conveys much of what we think and feel, they are produced by the facial muscles and nerves. The special senses of sight smell (olfaction), taste, hearing and equilibrium are all part of the facial structure. The organs for the special senses, the eyes, nose, mouth and ears, each have nerve endings called receptors, tailored to their special function.

The **facial muscles** also enable us to communicate verbally, in particular the lips, which help to shape the sound and air stream into recognizable speech and non-verbally by way of expressing our emotions. However, these muscles and others in the body are responsible for non verbal communication too, whether we like it or not!

There are seven basic human emotions than can be clearly defined.

1. Anger
2. Sadness
3. Fear
4. Surprise
5. Disgust
6. Content
7. Happiness

The muscles of the face are **skeletal muscles** (move and support the skeleton). To make an expression we move these muscles that lie **beneath the skin**. Unlike the other *skeletal muscles*, which are often arranged in pairs, have opposite actions and are attached to the bones and cartilage, (via ligaments and tendons - *soft collagenous tissues - ligaments* connect bone to bone and *tendons* connect muscles to bone), *facial muscles* can be attached to other (soft tissues including other) muscles and the skin. *Facial muscles* often have no oppositional muscles and the facial tissue they affect returns to a resting state because the tissue resists deformation (turgor). Skin turgor is an abnormality in the skin's ability to change shape and return to normal (elasticity). Some facial muscles can be worked completely independently of each other like raising one eyebrow at a time. Therefore, even a tiny contraction within one such muscle can pull the skin and change your expression which requires an intricate system of muscles and nerves.

There are **268 voluntary muscles** that contribute to your expression.

Muscles forming expressions are divided into **three main types:**

1. **Linear muscles** (share a common anchor) running straight up and down
2. **Sheet muscles** (run parallel, activated together)
3. **Sphincter muscles** (contract to a centre point) ring shaped encircle the mouth and eyes

It is useful to learn to recognise the various facial muscles in order to better isolate them, so that any extraneous movement is eliminated and the muscles used are those desired. Also by recognizing the muscles' shape, it is easier to understand how the face is moved by these muscles.

The muscles of the head that act on the face are divided into **two groups**:

1. Those that move the skin on the face – the **subcutaneous muscles** and
2. Those which move elements from the skeleton – the **masticators muscles**.

- **Subcutaneous Muscles**
  Move the skin of the face and not elements of the skeleton. They are distributed throughout the skull, eyes, nose, mouth and neck. The contraction of these muscles causes one or multiple folds in the skin always perpendicular to the direction of its fibres.

- **Masticators Muscles**
  Surround the jaw on both sides of the face. The four masticator muscles are divided into two regions and move the inferior **mandible** (lower jaw) and they serve to chew.

Epicranius
(Occipitofrontalis) (*epi-*, above, upon; *cranium*, skull - **the skull)**
Effectively it is two muscles the **occipitalis** and the **frontalis** united by an *aponeurosis* (layers of flat broad *tendons* - tough band of fibrous connective tissue that usually connects muscle to bone) called the *galea*

16

aponeurotica so named because it forms what resembles a helmet upon the skull; from the forehead to the back of your head lining up with the top of the jaw. Together they pull the scalp backwards and forwards. An example of which is to raise the eyebrows with wrinkles the skin of your forehead horizontally. You can feel it at the back of the ears.

- **Occipitalis**
  Are attached to the occipital bone and the mastoid process of temporal bone and are inserted into the *galea aponeurotica* a sheet like tendon.
  They pull the scalp backward.

- **Frontalis (the forehead)**
  Originate in the *galea aponeurotica* a sheet like tendon and are inserted into the skin above the eyes and the nose. The frontalis muscle runs vertically along your forehead covering the frontal bone.
  It raises your eyebrows and helps you frown. When it contracts it pulls up the **orbicularis oculi**, which creates frown lines on the forehead.

Temporalis
The temporal muscles are at the side of the cranium in the form of a wide thick fan. They originate at the temples and extend far back above and behind the ear. They end on the area of the lower jaw just below the zygomatic arch.
Contraction of the temporalis muscle elevates the mandible (lower jaw) opening and closing the mouth. Assist in side to side movement. Their action is primarily for chewing food.

The **two main muscles of the face** are the **orbicularis oculi** that encircle each eye and the **orbicularis oris** which encircles the mouth. Both are ring shaped muscles.

Orbicularis oculi
(*orbis, orb*, circle; *oculi,* of the eye **around the eye**)
This complex muscle consists of three parts, **orbital**, **palpebral** and **lacrimal** which together form a mechanism surrounding the eye.

- The **Orbital** part originates in the frontal bone and is inserted in a circular path around the eye.

It strongly closes eyelids ('screws up') the eye. Movement is around the eye.

- The **Palpebral** part (in the eyelids) originates in the medial (middle) *palpebral ligament* (attaches corner of eyelid) to *zygomatic* (cheek) bone.
  It gently closes the eye – blinking. Movement is up and down.
- The **Lacrimal** part (pertaining to tears) originates in the *lacrimal bone* (corner of eye by nose).
  This muscle dilates the *lacrimal sac* and brings lacrimal canals on the surface of the eye resulting in tears.

Corrugator Supercilii
(*Corrugator* muscle that wrinkles *supercilii* - **the eyebrow)**
Originating from the frontal bone, its muscle bundle passes up through the **frontalis muscle** to attach to the skin under medial half of the eyebrows.
It draws eyebrows in and downward, so producing vertical wrinkles and furrows at the top of the nose when they are contracted, as in frowning.

Procerus
(Long slender muscle **- between the eyebrows)**
Originates from **fascia** (strong connective tissue) over the nasal bone - the lateral nasal cartilage and its insertion point is in the skin between the eyebrows.
The action is to wrinkle the nose, pulling the middle portion of the eyebrow downward enabling strong 'sniffing' and sneezing.

Nasalis
(*Nasus*, nose - **the nose)**
These originate in the *greater alar cartilage* (tip of nose) and skin on nose and are inserted by joining the opposite muscle on other side of nose.
They produce the action of flaring and widening the nostrils. Their basic function is for breathing through the nose.

Caninus
(Canine tooth)
Originates in the upper part of the canine fossa below the orbital hole and it is inserted within the deep layer of the skin of the upper lip near the external angle of the mouth. The muscle shape is almost rectangular. It raises the upper lip overlying the canine tooth and moves the corners of the mouth. It can be moved independently, remember the Elvis curl!

Orbicularis oris {G}

(Orbis, orb; circle, **pertaining to the mouth**)

It originates in the maxilla and mandible, and its insertion is the skin surrounding the mouth and lips. This is a composite sphincter muscle unlike simple **orbicularis oculi** although they are both called **sphincters** because they contract to close an opening.

It consists of numerous strata of muscular fibres surrounding the **orifice** (opening) of the mouth but has a different direction i.e. it is attached to many other muscles. It consists partly of fibres derived from the other facial muscles which are inserted into the lips, and partly of fibres proper to the lips.

It is often referred to as the *"kissing muscle"* which closes the mouth and purses and puckers the lips when it contracts. It also shapes lips during speech.

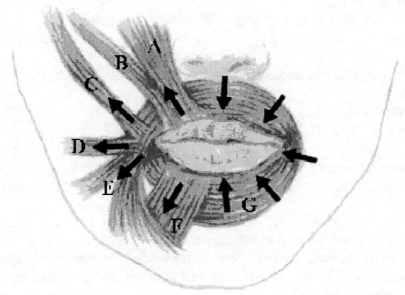

Structure of the muscles around the mouth and the directions of those muscle contractions.

A - *Levator labii superioris*
B - *Zygomaticus minor*
C - *Zygomaticus major*
D - *Risorius*
E - *Depressor anguli oris,*
F - *Labii inferioris,*
G - *Orbicularis oris*

Levator Labii Superiors {A}
(*Levare,* to raise; *labium*, lip; *superioris,* above)
- The *angular head* (inner muscle)
  It originates on an angle at the *zygomatic* (cheek) bone and the front of the *maxilla* (side of nose – upper jaw bone that holds upper teeth).
- The other branch, the *infraorbital head*, is adjacent
  Originating on the lower middle border part of the eye socket.

The *angular head* is attached to the upper lip and skin of the nose while the *infraorbital head* is connected to the muscles of the upper lip.
The action is to raise the upper lip. Interweaves with the *orbicularis oris* and lifts the lip. It dilates the *nares* (nostrils). Forms nasolabia furrows. It facilitates kissing.

Levator Anguli Oris
(*Levare,* to rise; *angulus*, angle; *oris*, pertaining to mouth)
It originates in a depression on the inner surface of the upper *mandible*, lower jaw.
The action is to elevate angle (lifts the corners) of the mouth.

Zygomaticus Major {C} (large) &
Zygomaticus Minor {B} (small)

- **Major** begins on the top outer edge surface of the *zygomatic bone* (cheekbone) and is inserted into the skin at the outer corner of the mouth.
  It pulls the corner of the mouth both up and back. Lift the corners of the mouth and are called the 'smiling muscles'.
- **Minor** originates on the lower outer edge surface of the *zygomatic* bone (cheek bone) and is inserted into the upper centre part of the lip **(labii superioris)**.
  It elevates the upper lip and forms nasolabial furrows.

Depressor Labii Inferioris {F}
(*Deprimere* - press down, *labbi* – lip, *inferior*- below)
Originates on the middle surface of the *mandible* (lower jaw) and connects to the skin of the lower lip.
The action is to pulls the lower lip downward and slightly laterally (outward).

Depressor Anguli Oris {E}
(*Deprimere*, to press down; *angulus*, angle; *oris*- mouth)
Muscle fibres are continuous with the platysma (in neck). Begins in the lower jaw and is inserted into the corners of each side of the mouth.
It pulls the corners of the mouth downwards to cause an appearance of sadness or frowning.

Risorius {D}
Arises in the *fascia* over the *parotid gland* (salivary gland) and, passing horizontally forward, superficial to the *platysma* and inserts onto the skin at the angle of the mouth. It is a narrow bundle of fibres, broadest at its origin, but varies much in its size and form.
Pulls horizontally on the corner of the mouth and is called the "grinning muscle".

Mentalis (relating to the chin)
This is the only muscle of the lips that normally has no connection with the *orbicularis oris* (muscles of the lips). A pair of cone whose apices are attached to the mandible (forward jaw) and the muscle bundle is attached to the skin of the chin. A dimple in the chin is the groove between them. Protrudes lower lip and pulls up (wrinkles, puckers) skin of chin, as in pouting.

Buccinators
Originate on the tooth-bearing bones of the *maxilla* (upper jawbone) and the *mandible* (lower jawbone) along a fibrous band extending from the mandible and is connect to the muscles of the lips.
Compresses cheek as in blowing air out of the mouth and caves cheeks in, producing the action of sucking, i.e. the muscles that are the substance of the cheeks.

Its action is to pull back the angle of the mouth and to flatten the cheek area. Also pulls the lips wide and tight.

Masseter
It's one of the muscles of mastication, the chewing muscle. Easily felt when the jaw is closed. This is a very strong muscle. Closes jaw and clenches teeth.
Muscles that assist with the side to side movement of the *mandible,* i.e. chewing food, it raises the jaw and lower the teeth.

Temporalis

The temporal muscles are at the side of the cranium in the form of a wide thick fan. They start at the temples and extend far back above and behind the ear. They end on the area of the lower jaw just below the zygomatic arch.

Contraction of the temporalis muscle elevates the mandible (lower jaw) opening and closing the mouth. Assist in side to side movement. Primarily they are used for chewing food.

Deep Muscles

Pterygoideius Lateralis (Lateral pterygoid)

(*Pterygoges* like a wing; *lateral*, the side)

The superior head of this muscle is sometimes called **sphenomeniscus**, because it inserts into the disc of the temporom and ibular joint.

Opens mouth and moves the mandible from side to side as in chewing.

Pterygoideius Medialis (Medialis pterygoid)

(*Pterygoges* like a wing; *medius*, the middle)

This muscle mirrors the **masseter** muscle in both its position and action with the ramus of the mandible positioned between the two muscles.

Elevates and protrudes the jaw and assists with side to side movement, as in chewing food.

Neck

Platysma

These are the superficial muscles fibres on each side of the neck and upper parts of pectoral muscle where it is inserted. Its anterior portion, the thickest part of the muscle, depresses the lower jaw.

When the entire *platysma* is in action, it produces a slight wrinkling of the surface of the skin of the neck in an oblique direction. It gives the expression of being startled or of a sudden freight. It also serves to draw down the lower lip and angle of the mouth laterally in the expression of melancholy.

Sternocleidomastoideus

(*Sternon*, sternum; *kleidos,* key clavicle; *mastoid*, breast shaped, mastoid process). Is a long strap muscle with two heads, the big ropey muscle that runs from the mastoid process (the rounded bump behind your ear) to the joint between collar bones and sternum at the base of your throat on the medial third clavicle.

This paired muscle pulls the head forward and down, and acts as a check rein to prevent the head from falling backward. The basic function is to turn the head to look over your shoulder. Example: raising head from pillow.

Further reading:
The Internet is an invaluable source of knowledge and there are some excellent sites to review I would especially recommend www.artnatomy.com

Artnatomy is an amazing fine art educational site about the "anatomical and biomechanical foundation of facial expression morphology." The Flash interface enables you to visually explore how the movements of specific muscles contort our faces into emotional expressions. The site was designed by artist Victoria Contreras Flores with text by morphologic anatomy professor Carlos Plasencia Climent.

Also, www.wikipedia.com is an excellent free encyclopedia.

Now you know where they are, it is useful to know what they are made, what makes them move and how they grow!

More about muscles - The structure of muscles

Structure of a Skeletal Muscle

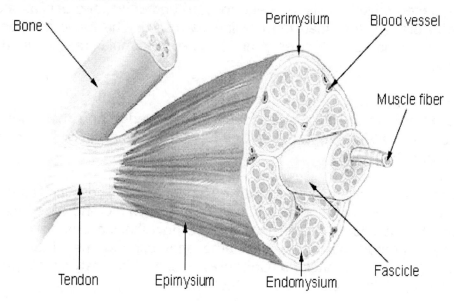

What muscles are made of

Each muscle fibre is surrounded by *endomysium*. The fibres are collected into bundles covered by *perimysium*. Many bundles i.e. the *fasciculi* are wrapped together by the *epimysium* to form a whole muscle.

There are more than 600 muscles in the body, which together account for about 40 percent of a person's weight.

The primary function of skeletal muscle is to produce movement through the ability to relax and contract in a coordinated manner. In humans **muscle tissue** is *contractile tissue* that contains muscle cells containing contractile *filaments* that move past each other and change the size of the cell. A muscle is a bundle of many cells called fibres. You can think of muscle fibres as long cylinders.

The face and neck is composed of **skeletal muscle**, these muscles are under conscious, or voluntary, control like the blinking of an eye. The basic unit is the muscle fibre with many nuclei. A muscle is a bundle of many cells called fibres. These muscle fibres are striated (having transverse streaks) and each acts independently of neighboring muscle fibres.

Each skeletal muscle fibre is a single cylindrical muscle cell. An individual skeletal muscle may be made up of hundreds, or even thousands, of muscle fibres bundled together and wrapped in a connective tissue (of which *collagen* is the main protein – 25%) covering called the epimysium. Fascia, is the strong fibrous *connective tissue* outside the epimysium, surrounds and separates the muscles. Portions of the epimysium project inward to divide the muscle into compartments:

- Each compartment contains a *bundle of muscle fibres.*
- Each bundle of muscle fibre is called a *fasciculus* and is surrounded by a layer of connective tissue called the *perimysium.*
- Within *the fasciculus*, each individual muscle cell, called a *muscle fibre*, is surrounded by connective tissue called the *endomysium.*

Skeletal muscle cells (*fibres*), like other body cells, are soft and fragile. The connective tissue covering furnish support and protection for the delicate cells and allow them to withstand the forces of contraction. The coverings also provide pathways for the passage of blood vessels and nerves.

Commonly as the muscle nears its end, the size and number of muscle fibres significantly decreases, narrowing the circumference of the muscle. But the **fascia** (together with the *epimysium, perimysium,* and *endomysium*) continues beyond the fleshy part of the muscle - the gaster- to form a thick ropelike *tendon* or a broad, flat sheet-like *aponeurosis.* The *tendon* and *aponeurosis* form indirect attachments from muscles to the *periosteum* (membrane that lines the outer surface) of bones cartilage, connective tissue of other muscles, or to a seam of *fibrous tissue* called a **raphe.**

The place where a muscle attaches to a relatively stationary point on a bone, (either directly or via a **tendon)** is called **the origin.** When the muscle contracts it transmits tension to the bone. The end of the muscle that attaches to the bone that moves is called **the insertion.** Unlike the body, the face muscles can be attached to the skin i.e. insertion into other muscles and *soft tissue.* Some muscles have more than one head, like the masseter with two heads, (imagine a Y shaped muscle, two points of attachment on one end and only one, on the other end).

MY <u>personal</u> theory on how deep folds and deep wrinkles form based upon my own extensive research

Fascia is like strong, fibrous, supportive cotton candy (candy floss) suspended throughout the whole body, connecting everything to everything. Overtime, this muscle covering web, (throughout which are nerves and blood vessels), can become increasing settled, fixed, anchored and semi permanently rigid.

Over time the *fascia* is adhering to one muscle more strongly i.e.it tightens to support one than the other. This forces the neighbouring muscles to pick up the slack, helping the restricted muscle do its job. Now two muscles are restricted and strained and the process of more adhesion and more restriction continues.

Fascia wrapping can also become adhered permanently to another muscle and will cause one muscle to stick to another. Therefore when a muscle contracts, it must drag along the muscle that is stuck to it, fascia tightens in the area to help protect the strained muscles and more adhesion develops as a result. Again the process of more adhesion and more restriction continues.

This is not a University PhD Thesis, so I will not bore you with the complexities here. But in my opinion, over time the *facial fascia* molds itself according to how the facial muscles are used. Personally I think, that this is what is happening with profound folds and deep wrinkles in the face i.e. repetitive action is causing the *fascia* to remember, adjust, tighten and fix in one place!

The *fascia* is acting in the same way that it does in your body. For example, when you cross your arms, you naturally put one arm in front of the other, do it the other way and it feels weird! You believe that it is your brain that has remembered, in a way it has, but it is not just your brain that is stuck in a groove of pathways, but also your insides, your body's fascia has stuck too! Since the muscles of the face are not only attached to bone on bone/cartilage (as in the body) but more frequently bone to other muscles or skin i.e. soft tissue, therefore my theory makes sense, well to me.

With **Fitface** facial exercises, by moving the facial muscles frequently and in all different directions the *fascia* gets broken down and when it rebuilds is not so rigid, becomes unstuck and rebuilds without the grooves and folds that it once had, so move those faces in every direction!

I daresay I will get tons of mail now from the experts proving me wrong,

Note: *Fascia* that wraps around the muscle is not the identical tissue type as the tendon issuing from the muscle, even though they are the same type cells.

What makes muscles move?

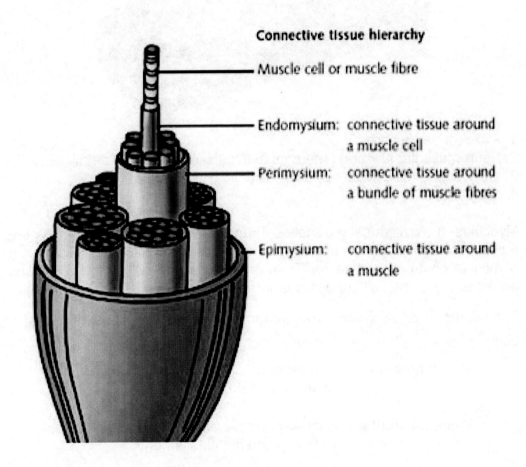

Connective tissue hierarchy

— Muscle cell or muscle fibre

— Endomysium: connective tissue around a muscle cell

— Perimysium: connective tissue around a bundle of muscle fibres

— Epimysium: connective tissue around a muscle

Muscle structure:
Within the muscle or muscle fibre are myofibrils.

Structure of Myofibril

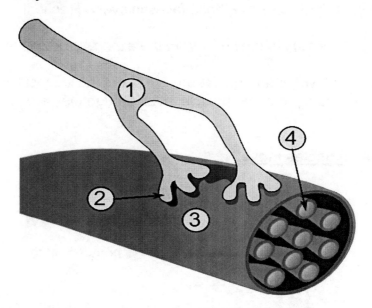

1. Axon (or nerve fibre)
2. Neuromuscular junction (see connective tissue hierarchy detail)
3. Muscle fibre (see detail opposite)
4. Myofibril

Myofibrils are cylindrical organelles found within muscle cells. They are bundles of actomyosin filaments (these fibrils comprise the mechanism of muscle contraction) that run from one end of the cell to the other and are attached to the cell surface membrane at each end.

The (*filaments of myofibrils*) myofilaments consist of two types, thick and thin.

- **Thin filaments**   consist primarily of the protein actin coiled with nebulin filaments

- **Thick filaments**   consist primarily of the protein myosin held in place by titin filaments

In striated muscle and myosin filaments each have a specific and constant length on the order of a few micrometers, far less than the length of the elongated muscle cell. The filaments are organised into repeated subunits along the length of the myofibril. These subunits are called sarcomeres. The muscle cell is nearly filled with myofibrils running parallel to each other on the long axis of the cell. The sarcomeric subunits of one myofibril are in nearly perfect alignment with those of the myofibrils next to it. This alignment gives rise to certain optical properties which cause the cell to appear striped or striated.

Movement occurs when an electrical impulse (action potential) travels down a nerve cell causing it to release a chemical message (**neurotransmitter**) into a small gap between the nerve cell and muscle cell. This gap is called the **synapse**. The *neurotransmitter* crosses the gap, binds to a protein (**receptor**) on the muscle-cell membrane and causes an *action potential* in the muscle cell. The *action potential* rapidly spreads along the muscle cell.

When a muscle contracts, the actin is pulled along myosin toward the centre of the sarcomeres until the actin and myosin filaments are completely overlapped. The H zone becomes smaller and smaller due to the increasing overlap of actin and myosin filaments and the muscle shortens. Thus when the muscle is fully contracted, the H zone is no longer visible (as in the bottom diagram).

Note that the *actin* and *myosin filaments* themselves do not change length, but instead slide past each other.

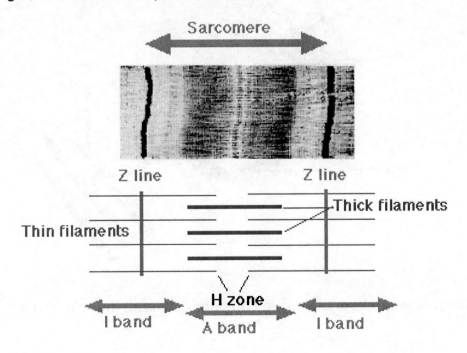

Diagram shows:

Sarcomere – showing muscle movement
- **Thin filaments** consist primarily of the protein actin
- **Thick filaments** consist primarily of the protein myosin

During contraction, the myosin thick filaments grab on to the actin thin filaments by forming **crossbridges** and the thin filaments slide past the thick filaments, shortening the *sarcomere*, like pulling a rope one hand over the other.

In skeletal muscle, the contraction is stimulated by electrical impulses transmitted by the nerves, the *motor nerves* and ***motoneurons*** in particular.

All skeletal muscle and many smooth muscle contractions are facilitated by the *neurotransmitter* **acetylcholine**.

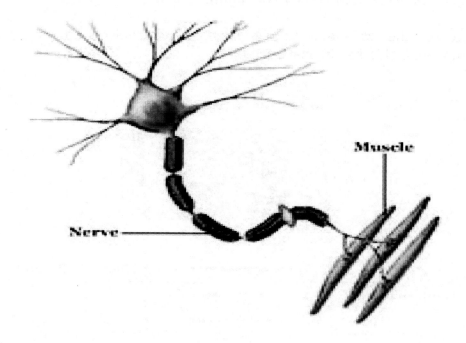

Illustration of how the nerve cell connects with muscle fibres

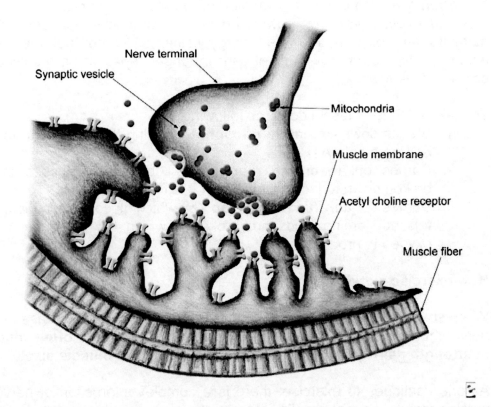

Nerve terminal

Synaptic vesicle

Mitochondria

Muscle membrane

Acetyl choline receptor

Muscle fiber

This diagram shows how the brain, via a nerve, communicates with the muscle and/at the neuromuscular junction.

(The area of *apposition* between the terminal tip of each nerve fibre and the '*endplate*' of each muscle fibre is a particular type of synapse called the *neuromuscular junction)*.

An acetylcholine receptor (AChR) is an integral membrane protein that responds to the binding of acetylcholine, a neurotransmitter.

The nerve impulses from the brain communicate instructions to the muscle to contract. This process takes energy.

Muscles are predominately powered by the oxidation of fats and carbohydrates, but *anaerobic* chemical reactions are also used. These chemical reactions produce *adenosine triphosphate* (ATP) molecules which are used as energy to power the movement of the *myosin cross bridge heads* and release the *actin filament.*

31

Mitochondria are a membrane-enclosed organelle found in most *eukaryotic cells*, the power houses, responsible for converting nutrients and oxygen into the energy-yielding APT to fuel the cell's activities. Without energy the cell can no longer repair itself, resulting in cellular breakdown.

To make ATP, the muscle does the following:
1. Breaks down - **creatine phosphate**, adding the phosphate to ADP to create ATP.
2. Carries out **anaerobic respiration** - by which glucose is broken down to lactic acid and ATP is formed.
3. Carries out *aerobic respiration* - by which glucose, glycogen, fats and amino acids are broken down in the presence of oxygen to produce ATP.

How exercise works

When someone starts exercising a muscle, there is first an increase in the nerve impulses that cause muscle contraction. **This alone often results in strength gains without any noticeable change in muscle size.**

As one continues to exercise, there is a complex interaction of nervous system responses that results in an increase in **protein synthesis over months and the muscle cells begin to grow larger and stronger.**

In simple biological terms, when you exercise, your muscles act something like electric motors. Your muscles take in a source of energy and they use it to generate force. An electric motor uses electricity to supply its energy. Your muscles are biochemical motors, and they use a chemical called *adenosine triphosphate (ATP)* for their energy source. During the process of "**burning**" ATP, your muscles need three things:

1. They need **oxygen** - because chemical reactions require ATP and oxygen is consumed to produce ATP
2. They need to eliminate **metabolic wastes** - (carbon dioxide, lactic acid) that the chemical reactions generate
3. They need to **get rid of heat** - just like an electric motor, a working muscle generates heat that it needs to get rid of

How muscles grow

I will touch on this subject briefly. However, I will stress that **Fitface toning** is not an intense aerobic or resistance training method. Your facial muscles were not designed to work at super speeds aerobically or to be stressed and stretched with weight resistance pressure. Yes, aerobic training is good for say the heart and legs; we were designed to run in the face of danger and yes weight resistance training when we had to carry children or haul logs.

However, that said I would like to begin, I'd like to cover the two main ways for an individual to enlarge the overall muscle size.

1. **Hypertrophy** refers to an increase in individual **muscle** cell size. The larger the cells, the larger the overall muscle, it's that simple. Muscle fibres hypertrophy = big muscle fibres.

2. **Hyperplasia** means that the cells remain approximately the same size but increase in the number of cells. Accomplished by splitting of muscle fibres in the interest of creating new fibres.

Note:
Although *hyperthorpy* and h*yperplasia* are two distinct processes, they frequently occur together, such as in the case of the hormone induced proliferation.

Human skeletal muscle undergoes **hypertrophy** (i.e. it gets bigger) following a resistance training programme. But is this whole-muscle hypertrophy the result of **fibre hypertrophy** or **fibre hyperplasia**. In other words, do muscles get bigger due to an increase in existing fibre size or an increase in the number of fibres?

It's a subject that has attracted/stirred controversial widespread debate amongst researchers. While fibre **hypertrophy** is well accepted and documented, very few studies have measured fibre **hyperplasia** in humans. Studies on animals have shown conflicting results.

I can only report to you what "I read, what I think they know!"

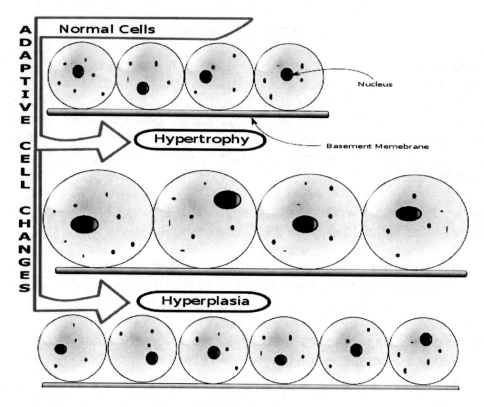

Illustration of the type of muscle growth:

Hypertrophy and hyperplasia

Types of hypertrophy

There are two different types of muscular *hypertrophy:*

1. **sarcoplasmic**
2. **myofibrillar**

- Sarcoplasmic hypertrophy

    The volume of sarcoplasmic fluid (the ***sarcoplasmic*** of a muscle fibre is comparable to the *cytoplasm* of other cells i.e. ***fluid*** of the muscle) in the muscle cell increases with no accompanying increase in muscular strength.
    Sarcoplasmic is characteristic of the muscles of bodybuilders.

- Myrofibrilliar hypertrophy

The actin and myosin contractile proteins increase in number and add to muscular strength as well as a small increase in the size of the muscle.

Myrofibrilliar is characteristic of the muscles of weightlifters.

Classification of voluntary muscular contractions

- In *concentric* contraction, the force generated is sufficient to overcome the resistance, and the muscle shortens as it contracts. This is what most people think of as a muscle contraction.
- In *eccentric* contraction, the force generated is insufficient to overcome the external load on the muscle and the muscle fibbers lengthen as they contract. An **eccentric** contraction is used as a means of decelerating a body part or object, or lowering a load gently rather than letting it drop.
- In *isometric* contraction, the muscle remains the same length. An example would be holding an object up without moving it; the muscular force precisely matches the load, and no movement results.
- In *isotonic* contraction, the tension in the muscle remains constant despite a change in muscle length. This can occur only when a muscle's maximal force of contraction exceeds the total load on the muscle.

Isometric exercise or **isometrics** are a type of strength training in which the joint angle and muscle length do not change during contraction (compared to concentric or eccentric contractions, called dynamic/isotonic movements). Isometrics are done in static positions, rather than being dynamic through a range of motion. The joint and muscle are either worked against an immovable force (overcoming isometric) or are held in a static position whilst opposed by resistance (yielding isometric).

Isometric movement

An *isometric* movement is a movement in which **no movement occurs**. An example is pushing against a wall, in semi motionless state with semi-contracted muscles engaged for a period of time.

Benefits of isometric exercises

1. Isometrics are purely muscle movements that place the stress entirely on the muscle fibres eliminating reactive contribution, and even so they increase muscle motor unit recruitment above and

beyond what you get from **concentric** (up and down) *or **eccentric*** repetitions.

2. **Activation** refers to the recruitment of the motor-units in a muscle. One can recruit nearly all the muscle fibres during a maximal isometric contraction – something that doesn't happen with regular eccentric and concentric reps. Basically, the more muscle you can recruit the more damage you can inflict and the more growth can occur which dramatically enhances strength.

3. Isometrics allow you to prolong the **time under tension** of an area.

4. *Isometrics* not only cause muscle breakdown themselves but also cause an immediate increase in subsequent dynamic work as well so you can perform an isometric exercise and stimulate strength, grown which can carry into your next movement. You can get stronger as the workout continues instead of having a loss in strength.

In an **isotonic** (dynamic) contraction, tension remains unchanged and the muscle's length changes. Lifting an object at a constant speed is an example of isotonic contractions. A near isotonic contraction is known as *auxotonic* (pertaining to muscle contractions that increase in force as the muscle shortens) contraction.

There are two types of isotonic contractions:
- **concentric**
  In a concentric contraction, the muscle tension rises to meet the resistance, and then remains the same as the muscle shortens.
- **eccentric**
  In eccentric, the muscle lengthens due to the resistance being greater than the force the muscle is producing.

Shot putters' do predominately *isometric exercises* whilst runners do *isotonic exercises.*

Isometric and isotonic exercises both build muscle

The difference is that isotonic exercises involve contracting muscles while moving the joints around.

Isometric exercises involve contracting the muscles while keeping the joints still.

You can find examples of both in yoga. That is what allows **Fitface** hands free facial toning exercises to be perfect for the face.

Muscle atrophy

Is defined as a decrease in the mass of the muscle; it can be a partial or complete wasting away of muscle. When a muscle atrophies, this leads to muscle weakness, since the ability to exert force is related to mass.

During ageing, there is a gradual decrease in the ability to maintain skeletal muscle function and mass. This condition is called *"sarcopenia"*. The exact cause of *sarcopenia* is unknown, but it may be due to a combination of the gradual failure in *the "satellite cells"* which help to regenerate skeletal muscle fibres, and a decrease in sensitivity to or the availability of critical secreted growth factors which are necessary to maintain muscle mass and satellite cell survival. In other words it is age related.

Muscle atrophy can be opposed by the signalling pathways which induce *muscle hypertrophy*, or an increase in muscle size. Therefore, one way in which **exercise induces an increase in muscle mass** is to down regulate the pathways which have the opposite effect.

Since the absence of muscle-building *amino acids* can contribute to muscle wasting (that which is torn down and must be rebuilt with like material). *Amino acid therapy* may be helpful for regenerating damaged or atrophied muscle tissue. The branched-chain *amino acids* or *BCAAs (leucine, isoleucine, and valine)* are critical to this process, in addition to *lysine* and other *amino acids.*

Your muscles grow when they recover after exercise, when they are at rest. (A-ha, so that is why I always look better the day after I have exercised my face rather than the day itself).

Without boring the pants off of you, *skeletal muscle* is the most adaptable tissue in the human body and ***muscle hypertrophy* (increase in size) does and can occur.** Muscle growth is a complex molecular biology cell process involving the interplay of numerous cellular organelles and growth factors. Strenuous muscle training leads to trauma or injury of the cellular proteins in muscle. This prompts cell-signalling messages to activate *satellite cells* to begin a cascade of events leading to muscle repair and growth.

This **disruption to muscle cell *organelles* activates *satellite cells*,** which are located on the outside of the muscle fibres. In essence, a biological effort to repair or replace damaged muscle fibres begins with the *satellite cells.* Working together **to form new *muscles fibres*,** often leading to increases in muscle fibre cross-sectional area or *hypertrophy*. This happens by:

> The *satellite cells* have only one nucleus and can replicate by dividing. As the *satellite cells* multiply, some remain as *organelles* (a specialised subunit within a cell that has a specific function) on the muscle fibre, where as the majority *differentiate* (the process cells undergo as they mature into normal cells) and fuse to muscle fibres to form new muscle protein stands (or *myofibrils*) and/or repair damaged fibres. Thus, the **muscle cells' (*myofibrils*) will increase in thickness and number.** After fusion with the muscle fibre, some *satellite cells* serve as a source of new *nuclei* to supplement the growing muscle fibre. With these additional *nuclei*, the muscle fibre can synthesise more proteins and create more contractile *myofilaments*, known as *actin* and *myosin*, in skeletal muscle cells. Confusing but true!

Influenced by hormones, insulin and *fibroblast growth factor (FGF)* is another important growth factor in muscle repair following exercise. The role of *FGF* may be in the *revascularization* (forming new blood capillaries) process during muscle regeneration, scientists are doing loads of research

Ageing, also mediates cellular changes in muscle, decreasing the actual muscle mass. This loss of muscle mass is referred to as *sarcopenia*. Happily, **the detrimental effects of ageing on muscle have been shown to be restrained or even reversed with regular resistance exercise.**

SUMMARY

There are 268 facial muscles, 600 in the body
The body is 40% - 50%muscle
Muscles are wrapped in connective tissue which is 25% collagen
Exercise builds muscles, don't use it and you lose it! **TRUE**
Many facial muscles are attached to skin or to other muscles
Exercise prevents muscle loss as we age, but nothing stays the same
Muscles are the underlying platform on which the skin of the face builds

All muscles grow by use, and atrophy when not used

Muscles need the right environment to build

Muscles grow normally strong - by having more cells, not just necessarily with inflated/bigger cells

Strong firm healthy muddles hold the skin on to the face tighter

Strong connective tissue is vital to look toned

Muscles are interconnected, tone one and you tone many

Isometric and isotonic exercises both build muscle

Isometric exercise causes muscles to build/lengthens by static resistance

Isotonic exercise causes shortening by lifting weights

It is so simple:

- **The facial muscles support and anchor the skin to the bone.**
- As we age the muscle tone and the skin *deteriorates* resulting in thinned skin and sagging muscles. Exercise promotes strong healthy muscles to hold the face firm.
- **The first line of defence is the muscles!**

Remember:

The skin is the superficial layer that **grows from the inside out** and it is the muscles that support the face.

Chapter 3

Facial Toning Exercises

General questions

The following are the general questions that I am most commonly asked. I will try to answer them without supplying a further chemistry or biology lesson:

What causes my face to age?

Ageing is a very complex subject that no one really fully understands. The fundamental answer is that our cells lose peak performance of functionality, our cells divide more slowly, and repair is slower. Our bones, bodies, muscles, organs and skin are all affected, as well as each different tissue type and skin layer, everything goes through many biological and chemical changes. In the vast majority of cases, your face, especially the outer surface of the facial skin is the visible reflection of your inner health.

What goes on behind the outer superficial surface of the skin generally reflects the causes that appear as ageing:

- **"sarcopenia"** i.e. loss of muscle mass, during ageing. There is a gradual decrease/loss of the ability to maintain *skeletal muscle* function and mass. The exact cause of *sarcopenia* is unknown. Most commonly shown in sagging of the face - where the skeletal muscles (which unlike the body's muscles) adhere (in most places) directly to the underside of the skin, are weakened through lack of use which become smaller and lose strength
- **internal abuse** such as poor nutrition, alcohol, or smoking causes premature chemical breakdowns not only of the muscles but also of the skin layers
- **external abuse** such as sunburn, razor burn, pollution, or excessive topically applied chemicals

In a nutshell, the muscle and tissue composition under the skin changes degenerates over time, leading to folds and wrinkles.

- The underlying frameworks of muscles which support the skin's underlying structure begin to deteriorate.
- At the same time the next major layer of fatty tissue tissues become depleted.
- The next layer up of *collagen* and elastin declines.
- Furthermore, the dermis or lower layer of skin gets thinner because as we age *fibroblasts* (*collagen* producing cells) become fewer and lazy causing the skin to become less firm, drier and even more wrinkled.
- **Elastin** gives the skin its elasticity, and *collagen* keeps the skin taut. Eventually both of these proteins begin to break down, causing the skin to loosen. The loss of elasticity makes the skin and underlying tissue more susceptible to the effects of gravity. Instead of springing back when pulled, the skin sags.
- The superficial layers also lose functionality such as the ability to slough off dead skin.

Accept ageing it is SO NATURAL; you cannot fight Mother Nature, even with needles and knives!

What are the first signs of ageing in the face?

The general signs are as follows:
- **loss of facial muscle tonicity** (mass)
  Ageing also mediates cellular changes in muscle, decreasing the actual muscle mass. This loss of muscle mass is referred to as *sarcopenia.*
- **slackened facial ligaments**
  Example of a facial ligament is the jaw (*stylomandibular*) ligament.
- **slackened facial tendons**
  Example of a tendon is the temple (*temporalis)* tendon.
- **depletion of skin's fat pads/layer**
  In the *subcutaneous layer* the fat cells get smaller with age. This leads to more noticeable wrinkles and sagging, as the fat cells cannot "fill in" the damage from the other layers. This is genetic and hereditary; there is nothing that **Fitface** or so called miracle cures/creams can do! If your parents had thin skin you may too.

- **thinning of the layers of the skin**
  Steroids hasten skin thinning according to Dr. Lawrence E. Gibson of the Mayo Clinic. Certain medicines, including topical corticosteroids, either used topically or taken orally, can weaken the blood vessels in the skin and weaken skin in general. (Do not use topical steroids if you can avoid them).
  There are some **medical conditions** that can cause the skin to thin; including Ehler's-Danlos syndrome, Frohlich syndrome, Cushing syndrome, Goltz syndrome, adrenal cancer, Cockayne Syndrome, Daentl-Townsend Syndrome, Fontaine-Farriaux-Blanckaert Syndrome, Growth Hormone Receptor Deficiency and Hutchinson Gilford Syndrome, just to name a few of the many
- **loss of facial bone**
  Bone mass shrinks, seriously, I kid you not - this does happens. Think of the shrinkage of very old ladies. This process begins beyond 45 years of age, however the good news is that women - more than men can be helped by diet and nutrition.
- **loose and less *elastin & collagen* fibres**
  The fibres unravel and loosen, which affects the underlying framework which supports the face of the skin, they lose elasticity.
- **dry skin**
  Skin without lubrication is more susceptible to thinning than well-hydrated, skin so remember to moisturise. If you eat a diet that is rich in lean protein, and additionally, you are consuming adequate amounts of calories on a daily basis, this will strengthen your skin and help it to repair itself if a tear in the skins develops. The skin's ability to retain moisture diminishes with age; the sweat and oil-secreting glands atrophy, depriving the skin of their protective water-lipid emulsions. As a consequence, the skin becomes dry and scaly.
- **slower healing of damaged skin**
  Cell division is retarded; therefore the ability of the skin to repair itself diminishes with age, so wounds are slower to heal.

There are two types of ageing:

Extrinsic (external) and intrinsic (internal).

Intrinsic (internal) ageing - caused by genes that we inherit.
  Natural ageing is a continuous process that begins in our mid 20's and the signs of which, are usually not visible for many years.

It is down to your genetic disposition; like the depletion of *collagen* and *fibroblasts* not working as they used to. Intrinsic ageing is unavoidable.

Extrinsic (external) ageing - caused by environmental factors.
External factors often acting together prematurely age your skin. Most premature ageing is caused by sun damage to skin, there are many other causes, such and rough treatment and the disease processes. You can do something about extrinsic ageing; you can change your lifestyle.

What are the primary causes of skin damage?

Sun

Sunlight is the primary cause of premature ageing. Prolonged exposure to ultraviolet (UV) radiation emanating from (called *extrinsic* or *photo ageing -* damage from) sunlight accounts for about 90% of the symptoms of premature skin ageing. Even small amounts of UV radiation damage *collagen fibres* (the major structural protein in the skin) and cause an accumulation of abnormal *elastin* (the protein that causes tissue to stretch). During the process, large amounts of enzymes called *metalloproteinases* are produced. The normal function of these enzymes is to remodel the sun-injured tissue by synthesising and reforming *collagen*. This is an imperfect process; however, to achieve it, some of these enzymes actually degrade *collagen*. The result is an uneven formation (matrix) of disorganised *collagen* fibres called *solar scars*. If this process of imperfect skin rebuilding occurs over and over, wrinkles result.

Smoking
- restricts blood flow through the capillaries (tiny veins near the skins surface) preventing oxygen and nutrients getting to the skin
- Increases production of an enzyme which breaks down the supply of *collagen* to the skin's structure. Collagen supply is vital to the skin's elasticity. It decreases with age but smoking cigarettes accelerates this process
- reduces the body's store of vitamin A which provides protection from skin damage
- inhibits absorption of vitamin C – a vital antioxidant for skin protection and health

Poor or insufficient nutrition
The intake of fresh fruit and vegetables that contain vitamins and minerals necessary for skin regeneration and rejuvenation (vitamins C, A and E), is essential without these the skin and tissues cannot perform correctly.

Rapid weight loss
Can also cause wrinkles by reducing the volume of fat cells that cushion the face. This not only makes a person look gaunt, but can cause the skin to sag.

Alcohol abuse
Not only does it cause rapid dehydration but also loss of important nutrients and retards normal chemical reactions.

Wind damage
Take a look at a sailor's face, most look haggard and worn. It is the combination of damage from low ultra violet damage and over exposure to rapid exfoliation.

Central heating damage/air conditioning
Caused by the unnaturally rapid, drying out of the skin, and i.e. dehydrating the skin.

Pollution and general environmental factors
Damage from air pollution, particularly ozone, a common air pollutant, may be a particular problem for the skin. One study reported that it might deplete the amount of Vitamin E in the skin; this vitamin is an important anti oxidant. Particularly ozone may hasten ageing by producing oxygen-free radicals. These are particles produced by many of the body's normal chemical processes, in excessive amounts they can damage cell membranes and interact with genetic material, possibly contributing to the development of a number of skin disorders, including wrinkles and, more importantly, cancer.

Gravity
Lack of, too much or poor sleep patterns; this is when the body repairs itself. Some say sleep lines.

Chemical injury
Such as too many cosmetics, acidic chemicals products, harsh detergents, abrasive treatments, fillers and surgery aid breakdown and thinning of skin.

Stress
We all know all about this and I am not a shrink. It would be a book in itself!

Drugs
Drugs even prescription interfere with the complexities of human chemistry.

So, if we are all trying to look younger; **what are we trying to achieve**, and what do we regard constitutes youthful, good looks and beauty?

The first part of the question is far too complex for me to answer here; it ranges in complexity from looking our best at any age – to - sadly forever chasing the fountain of youth, which is unobtainable. We will all age. Besides beauty is all in the eye of the beholder, however I think that most women would agree with the list I have compiled below.

Young skin/face		Old skin/face
Vibrant healthy	opposed to	haggard, leathery, wrinkled
Clear skin	opposed to	pimples, blotches,
Youthful skin	opposed to	(solar lentigines) age spots
Bright skin	opposed to	grey, dull, lifeless skin
Smooth skin	opposed to	dry, scaly, rough, pitted in
Glowing skin	opposed to	old, thick, red veined n
Unblemished skin	opposed to	pock marks, tags, flaws
Toned skin	opposed to	sagging, lax skin
Tight facial skin	opposed to	loose, hanging facial skin
Full plump cheeks	opposed to	sunken in or flat cheeks
Consistent tonal colour	opposed to	spider veins and marks
High cheekbones	opposed to	deflated/fallen cheekbones
Normal eyebrow line	opposed to	flopped/dropped/sad
Bright eyes	opposed to	dull/grey occluded eyes
Open upper eyelid	opposed to	drop/overhanging eyelids
Distinctive chin	opposed to	fleshy pouch under chin
No skin folds	opposed to	nasolabial skin folds

No frown lines	opposed to	grooves in between brows
Smooth taut neck	opposed to	folds, dips, & rings
Fine facial hairs	or	some dark whiskers!

What should I do to look younger? (In a nutshell)

- Exercise your facial muscles - they will tone up and lift your sagging face. As a by product, exercise will encourage the dermis, (or lower layer of skin, which is comprised of several different types of tissue, within which are the proteins elastin and collagen) to regenerate
- Exercise your body
- Avoid the sun and never go out without a sunscreen
- Eat a healthy diet
- Drink plenty of water
- Quit smoking
- Limit sugar and/or alcohol

What does the skin consist of?

It is the largest organ in the body and that is why it is so important to take care of it! On average, an adult has from 18-20 square feet (about 2 square meters) of skin, which weighs about 6 pounds (2.7 kg). Human skin is only about 0.07 inches (2 mm) thick.

The skin is made up of multiple layers (7) of epithelial tissues (these tissues of closely packed *flat* cells mostly line the body surfaces and protects other tissues from damage and dehydration).

Structure of the 7 layers of skin

The distinct layer types of the skin:
See illustration overleaf

1. **Epidermis** (top) contains skin cells, pigment, and proteins.
2. **Dermis (middle)** contains blood vessels, nerves, hair follicles, and oil glands. The dermis provides nutrients to the epidermis.
3. **Hypodermis (inner) (subcutaneous fat)** contains sweat glands, some hair follicles, blood vessels, and fat. Each layer also contains connective tissue with collagen fibres to give support and elastin fibres to provide flexibility and strength.

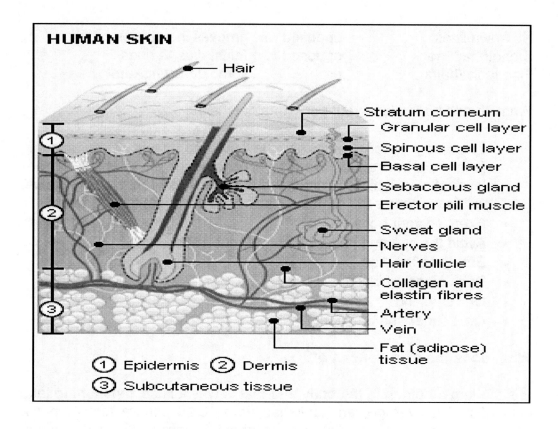

HUMAN SKIN

Hair — Stratum corneum
— Granular cell layer
— Spinous cell layer
— Basal cell layer
— Sebaceous gland
— Erector pili muscle
— Sweat gland
— Nerves
— Hair follicle
— Collagen and elastin fibres
— Artery
— Vein
— Fat (adipose) tissue

① Epidermis ② Dermis ③ Subcutaneous tissue

5 layers of the Epidermis **(top external layer first)**

1. **Stratum Corneum**
2. **Stratum Lucidum**
   (Only in thick skin, for example: like palms of hands and soles).
3. **Stratum Granulosum**
4. **Stratum Spinosum**
5. **Stratum Germinativum**
   (Or basal layer, stratum basale)

2 layers of the Dermis

1. **Dermal Papillary layer**
2. **Dermal Reticular layer** (the location of a lot of structures, such as hair follicles & blood vessels)

The 7 layers of the skin, along with the hair and nails forms the **integumentary system** (the organ system that protects the body from damage).

Functions of the Intergumentary System

The integumentary system is essential to the body's homeostasis, or ability to maintain the internal balance of its functions regardless of outside conditions. The system works to protect underlying tissues and organs from infections and injury.

Homeostasis implies a balance between cell growth and cell death. This balance is essential for the development and maintenance of *multicellular* organisms. *Homeostasis* is controlled by several mechanisms including apoptosis, a process by which cells condemned to death are completely eliminated. However, in some cases, total destruction and removal of dead cells is not desirable, as when they fulfil a specific function such as formation of the skin barrier provided by corneocytes, also known as terminally differentiated keratinocytes.

The skin carries out the following main functions of the *integumentary* system:

Protection

- Immunological surveillance and defence protecting the body's internal living tissues and organs.

  The epidermis serves as a simple mechanical barrier. This is probably the most obvious function for skin. Skin resists abrasion and penetration, and blocks the entry of foreign material. Immune cells of the skin stand ready to defend against invasion by microorganisms. Collagen of the dermis provides main strength to resist tearing.

Containment

- Protects the body from dehydration.

  Skin prevents loss of body fluid. Although the stratum spinosum is permeable to water, the epidermis becomes relatively impermeable in the stratum granulosum and stratum corneum.

Thermoregulation

- Protects the body against abrupt changes in temperature.

  The thermoregulation of the skin is carried out with the help of evaporation of the sweat glands and regulation of the blood flow to the *dermis*.

Sensation

- Communicates body status, sensations to the brain for action.

  The skin is the attachment site for sensory receptors to detect sensations of pain, pressure and temperature. It acts as a receptor. Skin receives several modalities of tactile information over the entire body, from a variety of receptors. The *cutaneous* (of the skin) sensations like touch, pressure, vibration, pain, cold, hot, etc, are felt by the skin.

Production of Vitamin D

The precursor present in the skin and UV rays helps in the production of vitamin D, an important nutrient of the body. When synthesised in the kidneys, *calcitriol circulates* as a hormone, regulating, among other things, the concentration of calcium and phosphate in the bloodstream, promoting the healthy mineralization, growth and remodeling of bone, and the prevention of *hypocalcemictetany* (disease caused by an abnormally low level of calcium in the blood).

Wound healing

Skin is extremely effective at regenerating after damage. *Mast cells* stand ready to trigger an inflammatory response if the skin is injured or the *epidermal* barrier is breached. Cells in the basal layer of the epidermis respond quickly to damage, proliferating and migrating to cover the site of injury (moving in under the scab). *Fibroblasts* also become activated by injury, to proliferate and to manufacture new collagen. When the *epidermis* breaks away due to a minor cut or burn, the cells on the lower layers of the skin migrate upwards as a sheet. When two ends of the sheet meet, the cells stop growing due to a process called **'contact inhibition'** (is the natural process of arresting cell growth when two or more cells come into contact with each other. Oncologists use this property to distinguish between normal and cancerous cells).Thus, the *epidermis* is sealed and the skin returns to normal.

Structure of the epidermis

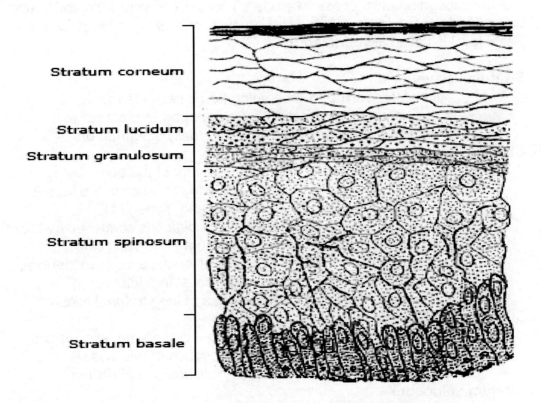

Epidermis {1 Human skin illustration}

- **Stiff thin layer of dead skin**

The epidermis is the outermost layer of the skin. It is made of several layers of *epithelial cells. Keratin* is a protein that makes skin tough and waterproof. The epithelial layer of skin is primarily protective. This layer, consisting of keratinised stratified squamous flat, *keratinised*, dead cells shed from the outermost layer of a *squamous* stratified *epithelium) epithelium* is tough, relatively impermeable, and self-replacing.

A keratinocyte is an *epidermal* cell that synthesises *keratin* and other proteins and *sterols*. These cells constitute 95% of the epidermis, being formed from undifferentiated, or *basal,* cells at the *dermal-epidermal* junction. Its characteristic intermediate filament protein is cytokeratin. In its various successive stages, *keratin* forms the prickle cell layer and the granular cell layer, in which the cells become flattened and slowly die to form the final layer, the stratum corneum, which gradually exfoliates. With age this sloughing off process which is 28-30 days in your 20's and takes up to 45- 50 days in your 60's. The process of making new cells at the Basal level is called **keratinizarion.**

Stratum corneum
> Cells of the **cornified** (becoming horny tissue *(keratin)*; synonymous to *keratinised*) layer are dead, protective *keratinised "squames",* and are eventually sloughed off.

Stratum lucidum
> Is a layer of the epidermis found throughout the body, but is thickest on the palms of the hands and the soles of the feet. It is composed of three to five layers of dead, flattened keratinocytes. The thickness of the *lucidum* is controlled by the rate of *mitosis* (the process by which a *eukaryotic cell* separates the chromosomes in its cell nucleus into two identical sets in two nuclei) of the epidermal cells. In addition, *melanocytes* determine the darkness of the *stratum lucidum.*

Stratum granulosum
> Cells in the granule-cell layer accumulate *keratohyalin*, visible as darkly stained granules. The presence of this layer is diagnostic for keratinised stratified *squamous* epithelium.

Stratum spinosum
> Cells of the "prickle-cell" layer are attached to one another by **desmosomes** ("spines") and reinforced by *tonofilaments*. These cells gradually move outward as new cells are formed from the *basal* layer (below).

Stratum basale/stratum germinativum
> Cells of the *basal layer* are attached to the basement membrane by *hemidesmosomes*. When a *basal* cell divides, one of the daughters migrates upward to replenish outer layers of cells.

The inner layer of the epidermis contains cells that produce the pigment **melanin**. In humans, melanin is the primary determinant of human skin colour .*Dermal melanin* is produced by *melanocytes,* which are found in the stratum basale of the epidermis.

Dermis {2 Human skin illustration}

- **Primary mechanical layer**

It is the functional layer of skin that lies just beneath the *epidermis.* The *dermis* contains nerve cells, blood vessels, and hair follicles.

The dermis consists of dense, fibrous connective tissue whose predominant connective tissue component is **collagen.** The texture of *collagen fibres* serves as the basis for recognizing two layers of the dermis.

○ The **papillary layer** of the dermis lies adjacent to the epidermis and consists of relative small, finely textured *collagen fibres.* This layer is named after *dermal papillae*, the protrusions of dermal connective tissue which indent the base of the epidermis.

○ The **reticular layer** of the dermis lies beneath the *papillary layer* and consists of larger, more coarsely textured *collagen fibres.* ("*Reticular*" means "like a network" and describes the texture of collagen fibres in this layer).

Like ordinary connective tissue throughout the body, connective tissue of the dermis serves several distinct functions.

- Tough **collagen fibres together with resilient elastic fibres provide mechanical strength for skin**. Lines of tension in the dermis, called *Langer's lines*, affect healing after surgical incision. (Cuts across the lines tend to pull apart, with concomitant tendency toward scarring, more than do cuts parallel to the lines).

- The ground substance of the dermis serves as the substrate for diffusion of nutrients and wastes to and from various other tissue components.

- Mast cells, lymphocytes and macrophages in the connective tissue carry out surveillance for the immune system.

- Finally, the dermis together with its associated blood vessels and nerves is capable of active response to injury, yielding the

53

defensive reaction of inflammation, followed by the healing processes of growth and repair.

Within the *dermis* are embedded several other structures, including *epidermal appendages* (sweat glands and hair follicles) as well as blood vessels and nerve endings.

The *connective tissue* of the *dermis* grades into the **hypodermis**, without a sharp transition or distinct boundary.

Over most of the body, *hypodermis* is characterised by **adipocytes** and may comprise a thick layer of *adipose tissue*. In some sites (e.g., "dimples"), hypodermis is fibrous and binds the dermis to underlying structures.

Blood vessels are generally larger in the deeper layers of skin, with only capillaries in the papillary layer of the dermis.

Subcutaneous tissue or fatty tissue {3 Human skin illustration}

- Allows skin to slide over muscle bundles.
- Varies in thickness.

Subcutaneous tissue is a layer of connective tissue made mostly of fat. It lies just beneath the dermis.

Skin Texture
Is affected the thickness and smoothness of the *epidermis,* by the quality of fibres in the *dermis*, and by the amount of fluid in *dermal connective tissue.*

Skin Colour
Skin is moderately transparent. Light which penetrates the skin is reflected back from varying depths by *epidermal cells*, by *collagen*, and by blood.

> *Melanin* produced by *melanocytes* and stored in basal keratinocytes contributes a yellow/brown colour to the epidermis. If the epidermis is not heavily pigmented, light readily penetrates into the dermis.

Collagen scatters light from the dermis without altering its colour. Hence, the whiteness of **white** skin is primarily a reflection of collagen.

Hemoglobin in red blood cells scatters red light and is responsible for the pinkness of unpigmented skin. The relative amount of pink in any given patch of skin reflects how closely blood approaches the base of the epidermis (i.e., how much collagen intervenes to scatter white light before red blood cells can absorb the non-red colours). Each of these elements contributes to the apparent colour of skin.

What is collagen?

Collagen is the main protein of connective tissue and the most abundant protein in mammals making up about 25% of the total protein content

Collagen is an essential complex protein (a biological polymer consisting of amino acids) that serves as a key structural component of *connective tissue* such as skin, bones, ligaments, etc. *Dermis*, the inner layer of the skin, contains large amounts of *collagen* whose fibres form a supporting mesh responsible for skin's mechanical characteristics such as strength, texture and resilience. *Collagen* molecules form fibrils that produce necessary fibres for our bodies. The configuration of fibres is the foundation for tissue formation.

As any material, collagen is subject to wear and tear: it slowly breaks down over time. Skin cells called *fibroblasts* are capable of producing collagen. When needed, *fibroblasts* replace broken *collagen fibres* with new ones. Unfortunately, as we age the skin's ability to replace damaged collagen diminishes and more gaps and irregularities develop in the collagen mesh. This process eventually leads to wrinkles. Thus, a comprehensive approach to wrinkle prevention and elimination involves reducing *collagen* breakdown and increasing its supply.

Collagen supports the skin, bone, cartilage, and blood vessels in our bodies. Think of collagen as a kind of rope, strong but very stiff supporting upright rigid scaffolding with elastin in between like a netting *elastin* acts as a rubber band, firmly pulling these stiff ropes of collagen fibre together.

Collagen destruction takes place as we age; 1% of skin's collagen is lost each year after the age of 40. At 20, you maintain skin firmness, keeping *fibroblasts* in place and producing lots of skin firming collagen. At 45, not only are critical collagen levels lost, but the *fibroblasts* that are still present simply do not work as well as they used to.

How can I improve my collagen?

Fibroblastic cells, which make collagen, are stable cells in the fact that they do not proliferate easily. **With exercise** collagen breaks down and rebuilds itself. Muscles and connective tissue are naturally equipped to repair themselves by producing new muscles and collagen proteins.

Professor Stuart Warden, Director of Physical Therapy Research at Indiana University, informed the New York Times (Sept 2009) that "**the stresses of exercise activate a particular molecular pathway that increases collagen**," which leads to stronger connective tissues in the dermis, and thus, fewer wrinkles and younger-looking skin.

STOP EATING SO MUCH SUGAR!
Sugar is exceptionally damaging to your skin because it attaches to the proteins of *collagen*, causing collagen to "**crosslink**". **When collagen cross-links it becomes stiff and inflexible leading to the wrinkling and stiffness of old skin.**

What is elastin?

Elastin is a protein in our body that is found in the walls of our arteries, in our lungs, intestines and even our skin. As the name suggests elastin gives our organs, elasticity. Working in partnership with *collagen*, *elastin* allows the body organs to stretch and relax. Thus, whilst *collagen* provides rigidity, *elastin* allows the blood vessels and heart tissues, for example, to stretch and then revert to their original positions. It is less abundant than *collagen*.

Our skin contains *elastin* which over time can be damaged by the sun's ultraviolet (UV) light. The breakdown of these fibres causes the skin to lose its ability to snap back after stretching. As a result, wrinkles form.

How can I build elastin?

Elastin forms between collagen which is 25% of connective tissue of muscle fibre therefore as you build one, you build the other it forms around it. **Muscles build, grow and stay healthy with exercise,** without which they together with collagen and elastin become weak and slacken.

What are free radicals?

Free radicals are atoms or groups of atoms with an odd (unpaired) number of electrons and can be formed when oxygen interacts with certain molecules. All molecules want to have a pair of electrons in their outer orbit. They search around looking for a second electron to complete the pair; they are out of control and damage other cells in their quest but appear only for a nanosecond.

Some free radicals arise normally during metabolism. Sometimes the body's immune system's cells purposefully create them to neutralise viruses and bacteria. However, environmental factors such as pollution, radiation, cigarette smoke and herbicides can also spawn free radicals. For example, in the processes of metalloproteinases (sun damaged discussed earlier) is the over production of oxidants also called *free radicals*. **Normally, the body can handle *free radicals*,** BUT if *antioxidants* are unavailable <u>through good nutrition,</u> or if the free-radical production becomes excessive, damage can occur. Of particular importance is that free radical damage accumulates with age. (If you eat nutritiously, well balanced meals, stay out of the sun etc beware, that the need for *antioxidants* to counter act free radicals is HYPE)!

Once formed these highly reactive radicals can start a chain reaction, like dominoes. Their chief danger comes from the damage they can do when they react with important cellular components such as DNA, or the cell membrane. Cells may function poorly or die if this occurs. If they take the extra electron they need from the *collagen* molecules in our skin, the result is that the collagen becomes damaged. When the collagen becomes damaged, the skin gets discolored and stiff and loses elasticity. The end result is that the free radicals sap our skin of its youthful appearance.

To prevent free radical damage the body has a defence system of *antioxidants.* However remember our cells use oxygen to produce energy and in the process they generate free radicals during such basic metabolic functions as circulation and digestion. Whether free radicals are wanted or not ridding yourself of them is impossible, because they are an unwanted by-product of daily living.

What are antioxidants?

Antioxidants are substances that hunt for oxygen free radicals, the unstable particles that can damage cells. They neutralise *free radicals* by giving/donating one of their own electrons, thus ending the electron "stealing" reaction of the free radical.

Antioxidants are molecules which can safely interact with *free radicals* and terminate the chain reaction before vital molecules are damaged. The *antioxidant nutrients* themselves don't become *free radicals* by donating an electron because they are stable in either form.   They act as scavengers, helping to prevent cell and tissue damage that could lead to cellular damage and disease.

Although there are several enzyme systems within the body that scavenge *free radicals*, **the principle micronutrient (vitamin) *antioxidants* are vitamin E, beta-carotene,** and **vitamin C.** Additionally, **selenium**, a trace metal that is required for proper function of one of the body's antioxidant enzyme systems, is sometimes included in this category. **The body cannot manufacture these micronutrients so they must be supplied in the diet.**

How does the skin grow?

From the inside out, internally, new cells are always being produced and old ones i.e. dead skin is constantly being sloughed off. (This is explained in far greater detail; earlier, in **Chapter 3**).

Where does skin get its nourishment?

The skin grows with proper nourishment (from the food – only nutritious food i.e. fruit-vegetables-protein - we eat) and oxygen both supplied in the blood.

Why are facial exercises good for the skin?

Facial exercises provide increased blood flow to the skin, thus promoting growth and the removal of potentially damaging toxins which makes your skin, healthier. Exercise builds collagen, elastin and muscle fibres, making your skin stronger and more elastic. Skin that lies on top of good healthy foundations glows from the inside out.

Why does the skin require oxygen?

For the skin to function properly, it must have an adequate supply of oxygen. Red blood cells carry oxygen from the lungs to the cells to produce energy and remove carbon dioxide. Exercise increases oxygenated blood from the lungs which helps to stimulate blood circulation, allowing the skin cells to function more effectively, receive nutrients and achieve proper balance, no matter what your skin type.

As we age, the oxygen level in our skin declines, starting as early as age 25. This decrease in oxygen can result in premature ageing, impaired cell renewal and hyper pigmentation or "age spots" also known as "*Solar lentigo*".

To sum it up, without adequate oxygen, the skin does not breathe properly and begins to appear dull and lifeless.

Benefits of facial exercises

Great skin

- **What makes great skin?**
  Great muscles!

- **What makes muscles strong and toned?**
  Yes, you guessed it exercise.

- **Why?**
  Because increased circulation neutralises free radicals and decreases inflammation, i.e. **Fitface hands free facial toning exercises!**

  Exercise tones facial muscles and increases muscle mass, to lift and support sagging skin. The facial muscles are connected to both the skin and the bone which forms a "cushion" on which the skin rests. By stimulating those muscles through exercise, the underlying cushion is plumped up and toned. If this cushion is worn-out, compressed or not consistent in thickness the skin will look sullen, deflated and lifeless, consequently not looking its' best. With hands free toning exercises the muscle mass will be maintained, at any age and it can also be increased.

Reduces the appearance of fine lines and wrinkles

- **How?**
  Dormant, undernourished, lazy, essentially relaxed facial muscles sink and fall with time by the effects of gravity. The overlying attached skin falls and sinks with them, thereby over many years creating facial wrinkles and folds. By gradually and continually working out your facial muscles your skin will not be able to fall into sunken grooves to form wrinkles because few grooves or folds will have formed.

Smoothes and firms facial tissue, reducing droopy skin

- **Why/how does exercise help?**
  It is imperative that you condition your facial musculature or your muscles will become slack and lax, with the result that the overlying skin will become saggy, baggy and crêpe like. One of the major causes of sagging facial skin is a loss of muscles tonicity (mass). By exercising your jaw, cheeks and neck muscles you will tone up your facial muscles, therefore indirectly pulling and firming up your skin. Directly stimulating your *elastin* (elasticity) and rejuvenating your *collagen* (support).

Promotes collagen production, giving your face the bloom of youth

As we age *fibroblasts* become fewer and lazy causing the skin to become less firm, drier and even more wrinkled. Exercise **stimulates** the microcirculatory networks that carries nourishment to the skin of the face and thereby indirectly influences the production of *collagen*. In other words, exercise stimulates the *fibroblasts* (or collagen-producing cells) in the skin, giving your face elasticity and with increased collagen repair, rejuvenates the skin.

Collagen is a group of naturally occurring proteins, the main protein of *connective tissue* that supports your skin. **Exercise improves circulation** bringing out the skin's natural luster. The increased blood flow to all areas brings back natural *collagens, elastins,* vitamins and nutrients, naturally occurring in the blood stream, to the dermis giving one a vibrant radiance. Improved circulation leads to a bright complexion and improved detoxification as debris and damaged cells are removed. In précis the skin regains its natural luster.

Relieves the appearance of daily stress, making the skin glow

- **How?**
  Increased circulation (from exercise) neutralises *free radicals* and decreases inflammation giving you a healthy look. Late, just like after doing any other form of exercise, after you have completed your routine, you will feel energised and acquire a healthy glow. The worked out muscles will continue to work, just a little more efficiently even after you have ceased stimulating them with exercise.

Increases personal confidence, self esteem

By learning anything new is an accomplishment. Taking ownership of your own body, setting your own goals, being responsible for yourself takes courage and commitment. By being responsible for your own health and beauty and not relying on somebody else either injecting poisons or cutting you gives you self assurance. Knowing what you know, understanding what the right choice is (although it is not easy) **but difficult, and yet, taking the right step/s empowers you**. Understanding the right answer, be it not a quick fix, unpopular in some parts of the globe (although not the 2 billion in China), makes you feel good about being you. By looking natural; naturally, healthier and more radiant than others of a similar age, **Fitface** will make you will feel better, enhancing your well being, self esteem and self-assurance. You will gain self confidence - every day (especially if you stop looking at retouched photos of celebrities – next chapter). You will feel great just knowing that you took charge, ownership and empowered your own self worth.

You know you can look fabulous at any age and avoid or postpone surgery by combating the signs of ageing with **Fitface**, I encourage you please, "Just DO IT" as 'Nike' would say!

Judge for yourself!

Here are un-retouched photos of me, taken by ordinary/friends people
By ORDINARY CAMERAS on ordinary days!

To follow

Aged 18, 25 and 54

Me - Charlotte Hamilton
18 years old in Jersey Channel Islands

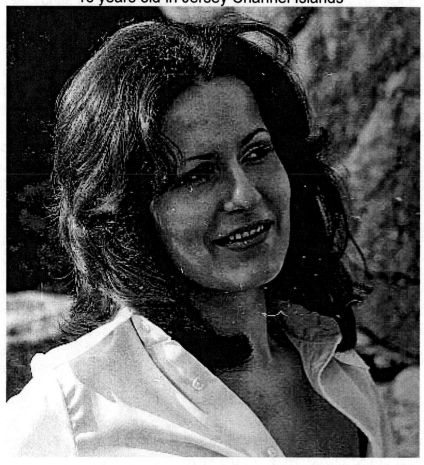

2010 Me today at a party at night (taken with a flash) - aged 54

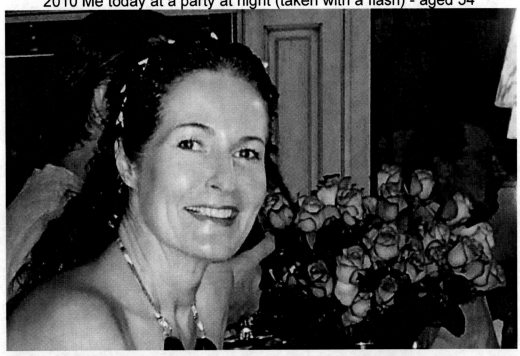

1981 California, USA - aged 25 - almost 30 years ago!

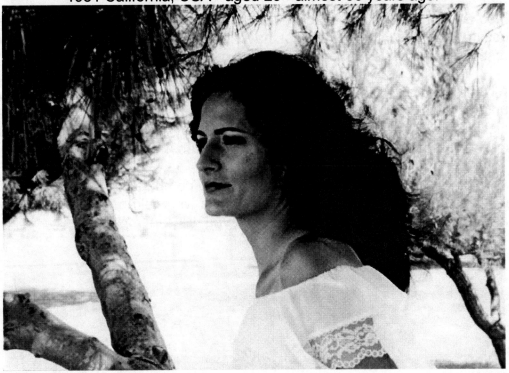

2010 Sunlight and windy - West Palm Beach, Florida, USA – aged 54

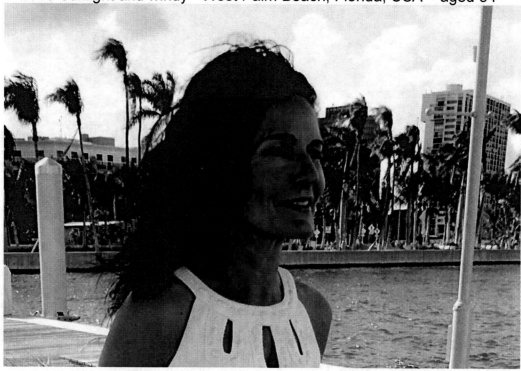

I too am sceptical of so called un-retouched photographs; so please let me assure you, that sadly I do not have the technical capability, financial resources or a huge name brand behind me to cheat!

All the photographs throughout the book were taken by ordinary unprofessional friends who were doing me a favor; none were taken by highly paid professionals. None were altered by anyone in anyway and I do not process the computer skills to edit pictures!

Are you still sceptical? Okay then let's do a comparison. Here are some of my "other body parts". These photographs were taken on the same day as I took the facial exercise pictures that you will see in part two.

My hand

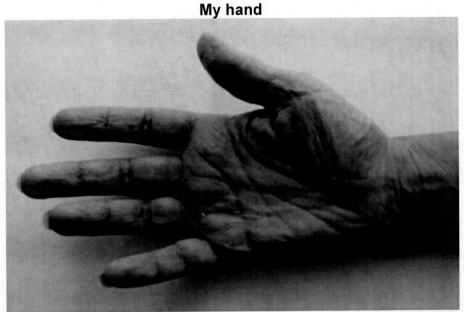

Below is the photograph that shows my friends' hand (to the right with the nail polish on) together with my hand. She is 4 years older than me, but my hand looks much older! I was shocked to see the difference. Her hand looks at least 10 years younger than mine! I guess I am in urgent need of hand cream!

Our hands

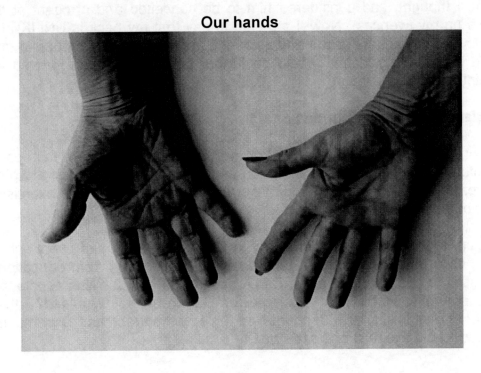

My elbow

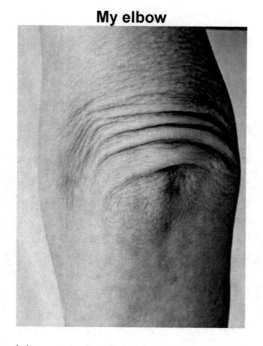

Count the grooves; I have 4 deep ones, and one forming! To this day I always remember that a hairdresser (of course whom I was in love with) told me that "he could always tell the age of his female clients by the number of rings they had around their necks, just like the rings of trees"! Um, I thought, and considered him to be conceited and arrogant at the time (in my twenties). Now, I am glad to say that my neck is UNLIKE my elbows, because of **Fitface** and it has the appearance of someone in their mid thirties. I could and would go further but I think I have proved my point, enough is enough!

Fitface's - added or bonus benefit

Your **eyesight** should improve or not degrade at such a fast pace. Nintendo DS has launched in Japan and now in the UK (under a slightly different name) a game to improve eyesight which is basically exercising the muscles of the eye.

Again, I repeat that it is mandatory in China, for each and every school age child (attending school), take time out (twice daily) from educational classes to exercise their eyes. Can a nation with over 2 billion people that are emerging as the next "Superpower", be so be so misguided? I think not. Strong/flexible eye tendons are able to contract and expand, i.e. focusing the eye thus one sees well.

Limitations of facial exercises

1. Hereditary conditions or birth deformities
2. Chronic medical conditions
3. Disfigurements by accident
4. Permanent facial skin damage:

   Fitface toning cannot remove skin damage blemishes, such as skin tags, age spots, scars or other permanent blemishes. Seek the advice of a reputable dermatologist and/or thoroughly investigate laser treatments. Verify the practitioners training and skill before undertaking any invasive procedure.

   If the surface of the skin is completely "shot", it will improve with **Fitface toning** but no amount of exercising can *totally* regenerate severely sun (or otherwise) damaged skin. Once again I suggest that you should seek a specialist cosmetic dermatologist professional for advice.

5. Reshaping

   Furthermore, **Fitface toning** cannot dramatically alter the shape of any part of the face as can plastic surgery; for example, reshaping of the nose as in a *rhinoplasty.*

Frequently asked questions

By far the most commonly asked question is:

What exercise can I do for this?

My clients say that, while pointing to a part of their face, most often the neck. I explain that, as with any exercise, muscles work in unison. You cannot go into a gym and point to your right upper arm and ask "What can I do for this?"

You must first understand and accept that the **facial muscles work together** like body muscles. In actuality more so, as facial muscles are not only attached to bone (as in the rest of the body) but also, in most cases to the skin. Look back at how the mouth works and the interconnections it has with several other muscles especially of the cheeks. Many of the facial muscles can work independently but should be worked together for symmetry.

I strongly recommend a visit to www.artnatomy.com or the link to that site from my website to understand more.

Fitface toning has been designed to work all the neck and facial muscles and not just one, although you can elect to include extra exercises to concentrate on your specific problem area or areas.

Are facial toning exercises new?

- No.

  Several facial exercise firming programmes have been around during the last 30 years, ranging from educational books to different devices. The advocates of facial exercises agree that if you continue the programme, the results will pay off. Massage and facial exercise regimes are preventative measures for stimulating muscles to keep the skin in place so that you can stay looking fabulous forever.

  "Ayurveda" is an ancient Indian science which uses massage and facial exercises as the key to delay the ageing process and help prevent wrinkles.

Are Fitface toning hands free facial exercises new?

- Yes.

  Fitface toning techniques are a new approach to facial rejuvenation from Europe. The significant difference between the "old way" of performing facial exercises and the new **Fitface toning** exercises are different to others in that **NO finger tip pressure is applied to the face** while toning. Personally, I do not advocate touching the skin while toning. With **Fitface** the delicate facial skin is not pulled backwards and stretched beyond its natural elastic limits. All **Fitface toning** programmes are **hands free**.

Do the Fitface toning exercises work?

- Yes.

  You will look more beautiful than you thought possible naturally. Exercise training works on the body and you can see the results. So too can you see the results of **Fitface** exercises on the face. Toning exercises are as beneficial for the face, as are body exercises for the rest of the body, no more, no less. Preventing muscle tone loss and increasing muscle mass, revitalises and rejuvenates your face; your muscles lift sagging skin giving you a youthful bloom. In turn this new glow and tone subconsciously also increases self confidence and therefore self esteem.

Will I notice a change in my appearance?

- Yes given time.

  Your face will look younger, refreshed, rejuvenated, firmer, toned and lifted, but as with all exercise it will take a little time and effort. It is not as drastic as any surgery; your face will not look pulled, stretched or scary just beautifully toned! Facial toning exercises are most appealing to anyone who is looking for a 100% non invasive, easy, natural, inexpensive, painless and risk free way to improve facial appearance.

Who can benefit from facial exercises?

- Any adult male or female above the age (I would suggest) of 25 years can benefit from the exercises.

  Fitface hands free toning training methods are for those people who have the desire to improve the way they look safely and naturally.

At what age should I start Fitface toning?

- I would recommend starting the exercises at the age that feels right to you.

  Your face will tell you. From my experience this varies from person to person but generally in your late twenties or early thirties or when you first consider buying anti-ageing products. I would be totally against anyone under 21 beginning these exercises as I am sure they are beautiful just the way they are and have yet to mature. Under normal circumstances I would suggest between your mid to late twenties to early thirties.

Isn't the damage already done?

- Time and time, and time again, I tell my friends **"No it's not too late."**

But they believe it is too much of an uphill battle to start. Any journey begins with one step. Those same people will happily spend small fortunes on the latest protein powder or a gym membership but talk about facial fitness to pull up those jowls or lift those folds and they have given up before they have even tried it. Wanting to do anything and believing it can work is half the battle and a positive attitude (like all things in life) is the key to success.

Am I too old to start Fitface?

- It is never too late to start **Fitface** or anything!

Survey after survey supports exercise at any age. That is why they recommend exercise for the elderly, to improve bone density and increase lost muscle mass. You will benefit. The body has an amazing ability to heal and rejuvenate itself; it may slow with age but it doesn't stop! Remember no cell in anyone's body is older than 7 years. However, obviously if you start in your 70's the amount of muscle available or its response is limited. I was flabbergasted that I sold my first book in Florida to an elderly gentleman Tom. But then I remember having just watched a You Tube facial exercise of a good looking man of 74. This only serves to prove the theory you are as old as you feel.

My mother of 80, yes now 80, after a diabetic hypo, broken rib etc, suddenly after a lifetime of being fat, she had a scare, and is dieting, currently – at the writing of this book – has lost 20lbs in 6 weeks. My point is - if she can do it, so can you! It is never too late to start.

What are the benefits of Fitface toning facial exercises?

- The facial programme will lift, tone, firm and strengthen all your facial muscles.

  Increased blood circulation will bring more oxygen and nutrients to the cells, i.e. growing tissues, while simultaneously carrying away damaged cells and detoxifying the skin, thus resulting in better tone which in turn brings back the radiance and elasticity of youth. Your skin will plump with the increased collagen and elastin as described earlier in the chapter.

Can Fitface toning facial exercises reduce the signs of ageing?

- Yes definitely, dramatically.

  Weakened muscles cause the skin to sag. Fitface toning programmes are a maintenance regimen to rejuvenate tired facial muscles by stimulating them with exercise, keeping them toned which in turn keeps the skin in place. It is not your skin that sags but your muscles that drape the skin over your face. Your skin will be lifted by stronger more toned muscles giving you a natural lift.

Could my lines increase with Fitface toning?

- No absolutely not.

  To prevent lines all the muscles of the face must be used not just a few. It is those few which are not toned that are showing the wrinkles! If you don't use it you will lose it. Muscles die, (atrophy) through lack of use. They need to grow, be strong, multiply. See **Chapter 2 -** Face and Neck Anatomy for further explanation.

Are facial exercises safe?

- Yes.

  Providing that your face is naturally your own! However, if you have had any injections, facial surgery or a major clinical peel I must insist that you first consult a physician before undertaking any of Fitface toning exercises. I cannot and will not take any responsibility for anyone commencing these exercises without the full consent of a physician. However, that stated in writing, my daughter who has had major facial reconstructive surgery assures me that she can do them all! See **Chapter 5** - A very personal story.

How do facial exercises vary from Botox or derma filler injections?

- Exercises are a truly non-invasive 100% natural, organic, preventative form of treatment, with no injections, no toxins and no surgery; therefore there can be no unforeseen reactions or complications.

  Botox is a drug made from a toxin produced by the bacterium Clostridium Botulinum. It's the same toxin that causes a life-threatening type of food poisoning. Botox injections work by weakening or paralyzing some muscles or by blocking certain nerves. Botox is a poison and prolonged use causes the muscles to atrophy from lack of use. Most injectable procedures cause discomfort (to put it mildly) and afterwards it is probable that you will experience some swelling and bruising which should disappear, whereas with facial toning there are no side effects. Results do not last indefinitely and you will either need to maintain a frequent, expensive, toxic regime of injections or have fun with **Fitface toning** which just takes time. With prolonged use of Botox or derma fillers the skin is stretched beyond its normal limits and requires increased amounts of the filler. Thus the face becomes increasingly puffy up eventually resulting in the new phenomenon of the childlike chipmunk face.

There are other fillers, some so called "natural fillers". For a more detailed explanation see **Chapter 5** - Injectables and fillers. Remember to ask yourself "Where does Botox go?"

What is the difference between a surgical face-lift and facial toning?

- Enormous - one is preventative, 100% natural and gentle lifting of all the facial muscles (forehead, eyebrows, cheeks, chin and neck). The other is a radical invasive surgical procedure with all the associated pain, scarring, expense and underestimated very serious moral, medical, emotional and psychological risks that only address a saggy face!

A surgical face-lift is requires radical surgery under anaesthetic. Generally they involve the removal of excess facial skin, with or without tapering the underlying tissues and then the rewrapping of the skin on the patient's face and neck. But it doesn't stop there. More often than not, you will have to consider a brow-lift, a forehead lift; cheek bone implants and an eye bag lift to address the whole facial area. **Fitface toning** addresses all these areas at once!

Face-lifts and other lifts are drastic, radical surgical procedures with all the associated risks. Has everyone forgotten this is not a nip and tuck; this is major surgery under a general anaesthetic, for no other reason than laziness chasing the unobtainable fountain of youth. They are for people who want a major change to reverse the signs of ageing or alter their unique look and are willing to accept the risks, pain, costs, complications and results of surgery.

Facial toning is for people who want a gentler, easy, fun and non invasive, pain free, organic way to maintain a radiant glowing and youthful appearance naturally. For a fuller explanation, see **Chapter 5** Facial surgery VS. facial exercise toning.

Research shows that 1 in 5 are more miserable after surgery than before (Ugly side of Beauty Channel 4 2010 www.channel4.com). Remember scarring is inevitable and if you have surgery "overseas/abroad" to save money 1 in 4 returns with complications.

How long does it take to feel the benefits and notice results from Fitface toning?

- Results vary from client to client.

You will probably feel an immediate physical change after the first session from using previously unused muscles and notice greater visible results as more and more time progresses. The improvement in colour and tautness in your skin is expected between 2-3 weeks based on an everyday facial workout. An overall fresher, rejuvenated and more youthful look gradually comes within 2 to 3 months.

Are there a recommended number of Fitface toning sessions?

- Yes, see **Part 2** for a fuller explanation

  Facial muscle exercises, just like body muscle exercises must be done regularly to achieve and maintain results. Little and often is the motto. Exercise daily for the first 3 months, after which do a **Fitface** training programme at least three or preferably four times a week to achieve optimum results. All and any exercises are beneficial, enjoy **Fitface**! Have fun and make it part of your life whenever it suits you!

What are the skin preparations necessary before Fitface toning exercise?

- Women should be makeup free with lightly moisturised skin. Men should be freshly shaven with lightly moisturised skin.

How do Fitface toning exercise techniques vary from the other facial exercise programmes on the market?

1. The major difference is that with the **Fitface toning** programmes there is no touching or pulling of the skin. They are all "hands free". There is no pressure exerted on the surface of the face to hold the underlying muscle. Personally I think putting any strain on the skin is a mistake. With **Fitface toning** the skin moves only within its natural boundaries of elasticity, it is not pulled beyond its normal limits. Therefore there is no likelihood of damage to overstretched skin.
2. There are no gadgets used in conjunction with the exercises.
3. I have practised them for over 20 years and have never had any injectable, filler, swelling cream or facial surgical procedure unlike the promoters of some of the other books. This really annoys me, it is so hypocritical. Furthermore, I do not take growth hormones, other chemical enhancements or use protein drinks.
4. **I am not a celebrity** endorsing a product just for monetary rewards, I do these exercise. I STRONGLY believe in them. Most celebrities will endorse any product if the price (contract) is right.

Good luck to them, I am not in that position. I developed these exercises. I want to spread the word and am fervently again surgery; cutting someone unnecessarily, for what? To look better? For how long? A few years? Then what? I do not see the point!

Why do some cosmetic surgeons and or dermatologists refute the claims of the effectiveness of facial exercises?

- Could it be self interest?
- Most don't thankfully.

How strange it is that almost all doctors, even cosmetic surgeons recommend exercise and good nutrition as the best way forward to optimum health. Yet when it comes to facial exercise they, the specialists are not always perhaps as honest as they could be. Why?

Most people would agree that in hospital, post operatively; the first thing that "they" (staff/doctors and nurses) try to get you to do is to get you out of bed and on your feet, even if you don't want to, and you are grumbling! Why do they do this? Because these doctors all know that muscles are self-healing and are able to grow stronger with practise and without use, they become weaker and weaker and eventually, they will die, atrophy.

The doctors know that exercise promotes growth, which is not bigger cells, but more cells by healthy cell division. This is achieved by improving the environment in which they thrive i.e. oxygen to do a process called respiration, diffusion, and osmosis (we all know that we will die within minutes of being deprived of oxygen). Nutrients are delivered, metabolism commences, energy is produced, and waste products are bi products which are removed. See **Chapter 2** - Face and Neck Anatomy & **Chapter 3** - How muscles grow.

So if all doctors agree that exercises are generally good for the body, why are dermatologists and cosmetic surgeons reluctant to admit that it's good for the face?

Cynically I would say that commercially and financially it isn't in any cosmetic surgeon's self/best interests to support facial exercises! Why bite off the hand that feeds you?

Medical doctors generally readily endorse **Fitface toning** and facial exercises, especially younger more imaginative, fresher thinking, and some more honest open minded plastic/cosmetic surgeons. The best quote I have was from an internationally renowned Beverly Hills (USA) plastic surgeon *"I do support the use of facial exercises. They work! However, I do many face-lifts when the age has gone past the ability of exercises to make the difference."*

In Europe many cosmetic surgeons recommend specific facial exercises (under strict supervision) following surgery for various types of face-lifts. Other cosmetic surgeons and others professionals in fringe related professions, may be unfamiliar with the various different programmes or techniques that exist within the broad category of facial exercise and are not fully aware of the benefits; furthermore **Fitface toning** techniques are new and perhaps have yet to reach them!

I have TMJ (Temporomandibular joint syndrome is pain in the jaw joint), **can I do Fitface toning?**

I am not a medically trained dentist, first consult with your dentist.

I am a slider, bitter grinder and have had many issues with my overbite and jaw clicking over the years. Most of my teeth have caps or have a thick veneer of composite. I cannot wear porcelain veneers until my bite has stabilised, which apparently will only happen with surgery. I have done **Fitface** for over 20 years without issue, but I am not you and cannot answer the question with any certainty.

Are **Fitface** face exercises isometric?

Yes, many in the traditional sense. Isometric exercise is a form of exercise involving the static contraction of a muscle without any visible movement in the angle of the joint. Isometric exercises are thousands of years old, with examples from the static holds in certain branches of yoga or Chinese martial arts (kung fu).

Isometric exercise is a movement in which no visible movement occurs; purely muscle movement that stresses muscle fibre. See **Chapter 2.**

Chapter 4

Celebrity Images

Self acceptance and the media

In today's Western society the media has an ever increasing power to influence, generate and sway public opinion. This is achieved through either editorial or advertising via the medium of television, radio, print, billboards or most recently the Internet. Advertising is designed to generate increased consumer demand for goods and services through the creation and reinforcement of both factual information and convincing messages. The whole modern civilised world economy depends on the consumption of more and more products and trades without which, there would be economic collapse with no call to produce or manufacture anything but essential food and shelter. Marketing creates our needs and desires for "*things*" that are ever increasingly superfluous to modern life. Don't stop reading, this is not an economics lesson, it is written to help you understand why perhaps yourself image is not as high as it should be!

Western women, including myself, seem to be especially vulnerable to the absorption of media images whether directly from advertisements or indirectly via celebrity endorsements. Advertisements are invasive, one cannot just ignore them and continual persuasive messages do get through. This is why they are paid such obscene amounts of money to support a product or service. Unfortunately, all too often we fail to process the media information correctly and we believe misinformation especially when it comes to pictorial or film images of celebrities. Female models and celebrities are transformed with the aid of; their makeup artist, hairdresser, stylist, publicist, other staff, designer clothes and almost always surgery or injections plus of course copious amounts of money, into being icons of beauty, fashion, taste and even intelligence. They can create a "fad", influence our morals and even cause international political apologies as we saw in the UK with Big Brother and Jade's outburst, for instance; unsurprisingly, making the rest of us feel inadequate, unjustifiably insecure and less attractive than we really are. We, non-celebrities, need to remember: **it is all make believe!** Sometimes, even the celebrities themselves get confused between whom they really are and the image they've created – we've seen the pictures!

I think it is very important for your self-esteem to feel reasonably content and confident with the way you look. The years have crept on me and I feel better about my image now rather than when I was younger. It's funny really, because then I was young and beautiful naturally! Perhaps because it is no longer so important or with age comes wisdom and self acceptance, maybe, I have just learned to live in my own skin. However, for most people growing old and looking older is a very unhappy process, hence the vast increase in unnecessary cosmetic surgery. Therefore, it is my crusade within this book to help improve everyone's self image. We all will age, it is natural, accept it and the more at peace with your own self you will be. Improve yourself naturally with **Fitface**, good nutrition, exercise, great clothes, going out, doing whatever it is that makes you feel valued and fulfilled by all means. The alternative is to spend your life on earth in torment, fighting a losing battle, with one operation after the next.

- **Accept yourself image**. That is not to say you shouldn't make the best of yourself and enjoy fashion, beauty and pampering, but stop putting yourself down. The most important lesson I learned was to look in the mirror and like my image. To stop constantly finding fault with my body and my face. As the thoughts still come in to my mind, I choose to ignore them. Practise. Every time you look in the mirror, consciously tell yourself you look fabulous and you will feel better, even laugh at yourself doing it! Laughter is also good for you. At the very least, stop criticizing and analyzing every conceivable flaw. Instead, **look at the "good bits"**, seek and you will find.

- **Accept that celebrity and/or model images are just that, images** only. We all know that most photographs are taken with special lighting, makeup, background and other special conditions. Even after all that trouble, if the image is not acceptable then it's airbrushed and/or retouched. Only then if it is perfect is it released! You know this is true. Put real pictures, when celebrities are caught off guard - on camera, of your chosen idols next to their publicity shots on your mirror. You will see a difference. Better still ONLY put up the real pictures of celebrities. You will have to remember who is who, as generally they are unrecognizable without all the paraphernalia!

Stop comparing yourself against fantasy images.

- **Accept and remember that most of the super star celebrities have had an entire barrage of surgeries, or injections**, to look the way they do, despite what they say! We have seen the before and after shots in magazine after magazine. How do they do it? We all know! It is one thing for a celebrity to advertise on behalf of a skin care manufacturer, it is quite another to have designed a whole skincare range and to **continually advertise a TOTAL LIE about how she stays young looking!** Do not buy into it. **Her image is not 100% natural.** It is **only** achieved by using either her own designer skin care line (retouched photos) or the brand she is paid to promote and/or by cosmetic injectable treatments, ("stuff beyond the reach of us mere mortals) or by the skill of her surgeon's knife! **Celebrities entire life, is their "image"** and give them credit, they spend 24/7 working at it and their financial lifestyle depends on maintaining the myth/lie that they project to you. One has to be a mega star like Sharon Osborne, or Kirk Douglas to put up with the enormous expense and constant pain. Even then, they don't always get it right, famously like Michael Jackson, Mickey Rooney and a host of others; even they are subject to mistakes and the laws of nature i.e. ageing.

- Remember all people **age is a natural phenomenon. No one escapes it** and personally I think some actors which have avoided invasive cosmetic enhancement are far more beautiful.

Unfortunately, for the most part, celebrities do not help the general public to feel any better about themselves; quite the contrary. The more distance celebrities can put between themselves vs. us the more idolised/supreme/immortal they become and therefore feel. There is still so much dishonesty among women about how they stay looking young. With a face as line-free as her young daughter Lourdes, Madonna says she won't "rule out cosmetic surgery. Rule it out? Who is she kidding? Bette Midler 64, (then 62), appeared on "Parkinson," a British talk show, looking fabulous and he complimented her on looking so wonderful. He didn't ask the embarrassing question we all want answered. "How does a 62 year old woman have the face and body of 30 year old?" Why? Because he is far too professional and knows that most celebrities are more likely to admit to having a drug addiction than cosmetic surgery. I could scream every time I hear the interviewer say, **"You look so young!"** <u>Enough silence celebrities</u>! You are mere mortals and age like the rest of us!

- **Accept that you will age**. Even though I strongly believe and endorse **Fitface toning,** I understand and accept that I am growing older and will continue to do so. I am pleased that I have aged gracefully and as with all people that are mature, I am thankful that I am fit, active and continue to be healthy. Those celebrities and ordinary folk that don't accept ageing and keep chasing the dream with one procedure after another become laughable, initially with taut faces like mannequins but eventually they look grotesque as if they were wearing their death mask, which I suppose they are.

- **Accept the way you are**. You have an individual look, a persona that is uniquely you, which is expressed in your face; the way you smile, that funny look, a worried look, it's what makes you, you. This portrayal of facial emotion was the first form of human communication, now with all the surgery and injections I think cave men would have a hard time understanding any actor. I especially notice the difference cosmetic surgery has made when comparing old films to new; in one I see naturally beautiful, expressive faces of the bygone movie stars - in the other are; emotionless, angelic, porcelain like masks covering the dull, lifeless faces of today's film stars. Rather than idolise them we should feel sorry for them having to go to such shocking lengths to remain popular!

- **Accept that fashion changes** as do the concepts of facial beauty and body shape. Think of all the trends: the pointed boobs of the 50's, the natural bosom of the 60's, the hippy look, the flat chested **Twiggy** ideal, the big boobs of 2000 - 2009 (once so in, now becoming dated), the big lips (pout trout) craze, the ultra, ultra skin and bones era. I could go on and on. Currently it is the "lollipop look" but as I write it is softening which means it is on its way out.

This is no longer of concern exclusively to females; the media is now influencing men through magazines. In my generation a man who read a woman's magazine was considered a sissy, today there are some printed especially for men other than Playboy or Sports relative. Even within the mainstream men's magazines 'beauty' crops up, even if it's just for Gel or Razors famously endorsed by a

British soccer star. Out of vogue are the dishevelled, hairy hunks of my generation, now it's the skinny, hairless, wimp, wearing moisturiser and donning the catwalk. They do not appeal to me but I am illustrating that taste changes and if you have had surgery you are stuck with the possibility of looking permanently dated.

Unfortunately, I got wrapped up in being a follower of fashion in the early 80's. At that time I had lush thick eyebrows all unfortunately they were not the fashion and stupidly had them painfully removed by electrolysis. For the past twenty years I have paid for my mistake by never leaving home without first putting on my eyebrows, with a brown crayon! Don't you follow in my silly footsteps!

Wrinkles have a profound impact on self-esteem. Indeed the stigma of growing old is evidenced by Americans spending more and more billons on cosmetics and surgical procedures. Perhaps we should pity celebrities rather than revere them? The lengths they feel they must go to, in order to remain popular and be in the public eye. The pressure must be enormous, but yes - I know, we would all like to be one!

Celebrities against surgery

Older celebrities say "No" to more plastic surgery

The argument regarding the pros and cons of plastic surgery, as an anti-ageing strategy is heating up, unfortunately more and more circum to the fashion and with them all the "wannabe's."

DON'T expect to see **Sigourney Weaver** booking a consultation with her plastic surgeon. The *Avatar* star, 60, thinks cosmetic procedures are unnatural — and especially silly if you're an actress. "I would never have plastic surgery or Botox injections," she said. "How can you as an actress? They both leave you with such a tight, unreal look. It's something fans and audiences pick up on instantly. Actors' faces should actually be able to move." And Weaver says she doesn't feel the need to go under the knife - because she finally feels sexier than ever.

The 64 year old British actress **Jacqueline Bisset** (Avon's spokesperson) has also spoken out very strongly against plastic surgery in a recent article, saying that she thought "Women who had cosmetic surgery looked like freaks." Even from the younger generation actor **Angie MacDowell**

81

(L'Oréal) has also been quite forthright in her views against plastic surgery - preferring to put her belief sensibly in a good diet, exercise and anti-ageing skin care.

Jane Seymour takes a similar line, despite admitting to having had cosmetic surgery to reduce the bags under her eyes. Hey, let's face it she was once married to a plastic surgeon so she ought to know! The 59 year old British actress has recently said she is against plastic surgery for professional reasons as much as anything, believing that the surgery takes away mobility and expressiveness in the face. *"When I see people on television and nothing is moving and their eyebrows are up near the corner of their head I think, how can they do this? They're destroying their expressions."* My sentiments entirely! Although, I must confess, she advertises her 'Natural Advantage' skin care line so perhaps her motives too are not entirely honourable. Besides I have seen the before and after surgery photos!

Advertisements for plastic surgery have bombarded the truly younger generation and therefore not so surprisingly there seems to be much more tolerance of plastic surgery among the younger celebrities and probably considerably more so in the USA than the UK and Europe. Despite this, several high profile young celebrities have spoken out against surgery including: **Kate Winslet** (being a celebrity rumours of Botox are rife but hopefully unfounded), **Rachel Weisz** (spokesperson against Botox for actors), **Diane Lane** (the face of Neutrogena) and **Twiggy** for whom I included the question "Where does Botox go"? See **Chapter 5**.

It's good to see that the topic is now up for public debate and that celebrities are beginning to feel they have nothing to lose by talking openly about the pros and cons of plastic surgery, just like the rest of us in fact! Perhaps things will change and the "knife generation" will be seen as a bizarre fad like padded shoulders of the 1980's?

In the meantime, with the realization that surgery does not work, even those stars who have been surgically enhanced are trying other things such as **Victoria Beckham** with facial exercises or more precisely Facial Yoga. Maybe she will change to **Fitface** hands free facial toning? That reminds me I must send her a copy!

Sad but true; I read that Cindy Crawford, Cate Blanchet, Julianne Moore and a few other truly beautiful women who are anti surgery have just given into peer (or should I say public) pressure and have had (only.... I hope) Botox, or could this be me being manipulated by the media and even this is untrue?

SUMMARY

- Celebrities do lie. Change their minds, are one day anti surgery and the next day endorsing it, "C'est la vie!"
- Understand that their lives, career, self esteem, world market desirability all depends on their persona and more importantly these days, their appearance. You know this; you recognise this, so take everything in consideration when you think about how "WONDERFUL" they look. See them as human too! They, like us, eat, sleep, drink and cry. Their world depends on us; we are the judge, jury and executioner.
- Celebrities' business/whole life is **all about** looking good.
- You are not a celebrity (or you too – or rather your "Personal Assistant" - would have telephoned me for a personal consultation rather than actually reading this book. Sorry celebs, I am not knocking you - you know the game – hey "Yes, I will take your jet anytime to visit you" – and more importantly, "Yes, I could teach tell you about the benefits of **Fitface** and teach you (or teach your personal trainer - how to teach you)." In the interests of protocol, our meeting - will of course be confidential. I am a person of my word, (see **Chapter 11** - Endorsements re famous plastic surgeons. Perhaps I sound too bias but I admire the celebs *spirit* and "gung ho" (positive) attitude. I was one once myself, be it only for 15 minutes; well, to be fair to myself - actually for a couple of years! Yes, I even had a celebrity date with **Piers Mogan**!!!! Now the "Britain's Got Talent" TV show judge etc. Lucky me? No ladies, I was not impressed. His uncle, (whom I met recently – late 2010) was far more courteous!

Chapter 5

Facial Surgery and Alternatives

Anti-ageing alternatives to facial exercises

I have researched tirelessly about the subject of facial exercises on the Internet as well as speaking to many UK and USA based surgeons and other professionals with a vested interest in beauty applications. The opinions on the best way to treat natural ageing varies dramatically depending on the prospective financial rewards of the parties concerned, be they by dermatologists promoting skincare products, medical doctors encouraging exercise and vitamins, plastic/cosmetic surgeons encouraging surgery, sports/exercise trainers endorsing natural exercise preventative methods or beauticians/estheticians supplying therapies/lasers and injectables. All understandably choose the remedy with which they are most familiar with and proficient in, which also pays the bills!

Age has also been a major factor in the attitude towards the benefits of facial exercise and toning. In general the younger the person I spoke to, whether in one of the above professions or a member of the general public, the more open and receptive to change they were. As "newer" children, then teenagers, these younger adults have been exposed to the benefits of nutrition and exercise. They possessed fresher information; consequently almost all thought that facial toning was great, most especially as if they had been exposed to the results of needles or knives on their parents. Those that were in a competing professions, added that they hoped that one day we could ALL work together and attack anti-aging on all fronts!

The older generations however were more often than not, stuck in their old ways and had not progressed with current knowledge and could be reluctant to listen to change. But oddly enough, all the young American girls and boys thought false breasts were a must. Hey, we all have double standards!

Yes, exercise takes time, effort and commitment - doesn't everything worthwhile? There are alternative choices available; some are radical "**quick fixes**", (with risks and expense) a few less invasive and <u>most</u> others fall into the feel good factor. For me, surgery is like having a tummy tuck when you should go on a diet and injections are like wearing those terrible girdles (when you should lose weight) plus 10 times the pain, risk, discomfort and expense. Besides they never really work or look natural.

I will take a moment to write briefly in this chapter about the ever more popular alternative procedures and my personal perceptions of these:

- Knife - Face-lifts & cosmetic surgery (see more later **in Chapter 5** Facial surgery vs.facial exercises)
- Creams
- Cosmeceuticals
- Super facials – combining techniques
- Injectables and fillers
- Resurfacing techniques
- Lasers
- Devices
- Spa treatments
- Growth hormone
- Weird and wacky (well, considered so in 2010)!

Face-lifts & cosmetic surgery

They are all packaged differently with confusing names that all describe a face-lift, here are some names:

- Macs Face Lift
- Mid Face Lift
- Endoscopic Face Lift
- Feather Lift, Thread Lift
- Subperiosteal Face Lift
- Temporal Mid Cheek Face Lift
- Quick Lift
- S Face Lift
- Life Style Face Lift
- Ribbon Neck Lift
- Weekend Face Lift
- Lunch Time Lift
- Mini-lift
- Deep Plane or S-lift

Plus all the other surgical procedures such as:

Blepharoplasty (also called eye lift or eyelid lift surgery). This is the most common in North America to remove under eye bags

Browplasty (*brow lift* also called a *forehead lift*). There are a number of different surgical approaches to brow elevation is large and include:

- **Endoscopic forehead lift**, in which the forehead is loosened and elevated through small incisions in the scalp using of instrument called an "endoscope"
- **Temporal lift**, in which the incision is made over the temple and only the outer portion of the brow is lifted
- **Midforehead lift**, in which the incision is placed within a deep wrinkle on the middle of the forehead
- **Direct brow lift**, in which the incision is made just above the eyebrow hair
- **Internal brow lift**, in which the brow is stabilised through the upper blepharoplasty incision (see photo links below)
- **Non-incisional RF heating**, in which radiofrequency energy applied to the skin of the forehead and temple supposedly tighten the deeper tissues
- **Cable brow lift**, in which thick suture placed deep below the skin mechanically connects the eyebrow to tissues below the scalp to create a suspension
- **Coronal forehead lift**, in which the scalp is incised from ear to ear over the top of the head

Implants: such as cheek, jaw or chin and all other purely aesthetic facial surgical procedures.

Should this be considered an alternative to **Fitface** facial toning exercises? **No**, not by me, however there are other people who will consider it so, therefore I shall include it as an alternative. That is, because the general public wants a quick fix option to **Fitface** facial toning exercises, a choice – especially when they have a readily available disposable income but are time poor. Regrettably the pain and suffering, associated real risks and side effects seem to vanish into insignificance after a consultation with a distinguished cosmetic surgeon who tells them how dreadful they look but how wonderful they could look and feel after surgery. Flattery will get you everywhere! Cynical? Yes!

Cosmetic surgeons **sell dreams**. Some even turn it into an opportunity and advertise "Make your dreams come true." "Be the best you can." Now, let's be honest here. "Look the best money can buy" (providing everything goes to plan and you don't over spend or if you don't spend enough, you will look like a freak). They brush over the pain, skim through potential side effects and don't even know themselves what unforeseen allergic reactions or complications can sometimes arise from cosmetic surgery. They certainly would not dream about lecturing you on the possibility of death resulting from the anaesthetic or pulmonary problems, let alone elaborating on any complications which could occur at a surgeon's office to an outpatient which may result in death. Tragically, they do occur, such was the fate of an 18 year old in March of 2008 in Boca Raton, Florida, who died after corrective breast surgery.

Surprising these well informed intelligent ladies aged between 20 and 70 have even accepted that (as a matter of course) the results of any face-lift are not permanent. That fact is no longer hidden under the carpet but openly discussed pre surgery. The client knows that they will always need another face-lift! A replicated performance, further explained risks, repeated pain and suffering and more money! They are also told that a face-lift is just for sagging skin and that other "lifts" are available to deal with all the other areas of concern like an eyebrow lift or forehead lift. There are also given the opportunity to purchase implants to put in their cheeks and or chin, where nature never intended them to be, for a totally rejuvenated look. Finally, they are even told that post surgery the skin will be less elastic and thinner from being stretched!

There is sufficient information available (for those that want to know) about facial surgery, both good and bad. Therefore, we should all understand the facts by now. So why do the majority of people still delude themselves into still believing surgery is a nip and tuck? I assume it is the power of the media and simply convenience and pain versus time and energy? However, I will concede that eventually there does come a time in very old age past where the ability of exercises to make a difference is marginal but by then, there are probably more pressing health concerns to worry about anyway.

I am not a physician, therefore I do not feel adequately qualified to give you more than a lay person's personal opinion on what I feel and think, although I have done considerably more research during the course of writing this book, and have had more personal experiences with cosmetic surgery during my lifetime than the average person. Whether major or minor, upper or lower face-lifts, involving the muscles or not, are beneficial or not; depend on one's personal perspective. Your satisfaction or not, depends on how, why and what lift or lifts you select and the skill of the surgeon who performs your operation/s and most importantly your expectations.

Surgery can only stretch and pull up droopy skin and/or muscles to give your face a tight mannequin perfect face for a short period of time in your life but it does not arrest the ageing process. Face-lifts vary enormously; they can look wonderful initially, just like the hide on a new pair of chamois leather shoes. However in no time at all, the skin, like the shoes becomes stretched and therefore is thinner than before with correspondingly less natural elasticity and the skin is unable to return to its previous state. A little like stretching a rubber band, cutting off a little bit and then trying to stretch it back to the original size. With each progressive face-lift (we all know that they last less than 10 years), you have less and less raw material to work with. Therefore with each successive face-lift the skin becomes thinner and tighter, the recipient consequently requiring a face-lift sooner, a vicious circle ensues - until eventually, the supreme **wind tunnel effect** is created, in a sad but captivating effort to turn back the clock.

In my opinion a face-lift only for vanity's sake, is not only painful but also a costly form of self mutilation. However **the choice is yours**. For me; an anti-ageing preventative method is better than cure. Facial toning addresses the whole face, but I kid you not, it does take time and the results are not as dramatic in the short term. Practise makes perfect, just as it does when you go to the gym for your body, results show.

I repeat that what I have already written: the results of face-lifts unfortunately do not last more than ten years, regrettably they are often not always good in the first place and they carry the additional risk that sometimes you can come out looking worse than when you went in! Building facial muscles lasts forever. However, the most disturbing fact is that when the next face-lift is required, the results will last even less time than before, therefore giving you a diminishing rate of return. Henceforth, sadly one does become less satisfied with each lift, while continually ageing and desiring even more than before. Knowing that one can always buy another face-lift encourages repetition of the never ending cycle of surgery.

Creams (see how the skin works earlier in **Fitface Chapter 3**)

I have read books and books on the subject of skin of "how it works", "how it grows and what nourishes it." These were all written by the world's foremost authorities, all looking for the answer to ageing skin, and I can assure you that anti-ageing creams do not lift or tone sagging muscles. They are a superficial treatment. They hydrate the skin. Some nourish and therefore definitely improve the texture, tone and smoothness of your skin. A few of the latest creams are designed to penetrate deeper and plump up the skin to diminish tiny wrinkles, while others have an ingredient to tighten the skin, however they cannot possibly "lift" the face to any significant degree.

Quality moisturisers act in the same way; hydrating the skin, with some having the additional benefit of protection against damaging UV rays. Creams, lotions and potions with regular beautician visits do have a feel good factor. So, go ahead, spoil yourself, if you think they will make you look better - then they probably will! Although, I would advise caution as you do not want to overload your skin with too many products. Find something that works for you and stick with it.

Cosmeceuticals

Your skin grows and is constantly renewing itself <u>from the bottom up, from the inside out</u>. Remember that and you won't go far wrong.

There are new brands of technologically advanced creams on the market with all sorts of claims. It is a multibillion dollar market and the winner takes all. I have read many reports some bad, some okay and surprisingly some good by well respected beauty journalists. Wouldn't it be wonderful if there was something that really did work? I still find it impossible to believe how this could work as these are superficial treatments. How far can and should creams penetrate the skin which has seven layers and then, what could they do except very marginally perhaps firm or plump? The largest organ in the body was designed as a barrier to keep dirt and bacteria out and not to let things in.

Cosmetics don't have to be FDA approved to be sold and registering them is voluntary. Cosmetics do not have to be effective, just safe to be marketed. Only when a company claims that its product affects the structure or function of the body is it then classified as a drug. If skin creams actually did what they claim – wrinkle and stretch mark reduction, stimulation of collagen or formation thereof etc they would then need to be classified as a drug and only available on prescription. That too can lead to a problem, as most people do understand that the sales girl at a department store will try to sell them the most expensive product but trust their doctor to prescribe what is right for them, regardless of bottom line profitability. If your doctor recommends a particular cream for your skin, he should have read the literature and be able to quote studies demonstrating the effectiveness of the drug. It is impossible even for a physician, to independently know whether a cream is effective without proof, **so ask for proof!**

Creams may work well in the laboratory test tube but do not always work topically (on the skin) in the same manner. Some cannot even penetrate through the various layers of the skin to be effective (despite the advertising campaigns). Imagine your skin as a chain link fence, some creams will go through, others won't. It all depends on the size of the molecules in the cream. Large molecules such as growth hormones, proteins, *collagen* and *hyaluronic acid* have little chance of penetrating the skin. For example *Botox* is injected into the skin through the fence to alleviate that problem. Glycolic acid, Vit C and *tretinoin* pass through. *Peptides* are impressive in the test tube but the big question is whether the large molecules can penetrate the skin and cause real change.

I am trying to stop you from wasting your money on the many products on the market that contain *collagen* and make great claims – **they don't work!** I know this is counter-intuitive; if your skin needs to rebuild *collagen* and **the product contains *collagen*, must work, right? Well, no.** The reason these collagen-containing products don't work is that the collagen **molecules are just too large/big** to get inside the skin and do their job of rebuilding. In short, they are simply imposters.

Despite what the packages may say, creams containing collagen work on the skin's surface only and cannot reverse the effects of collagen loss, which occurs deep in the skin's layers. Instead, these creams work to prevent the loss of moisture on the skin's surface, which keeps its appearance smooth.

The packaging and promotion of skin care creams is simply amazing, especially the newer anti-ageing products. Much, of it for me is extremely misleading, the mind boggles. Among the new generation of creams are those that claim allegiance to stem cell technology, arising from stem cell research with a unique ability to protect the skin from further damage and deterioration. Well that's the blurb but it simply cannot stop the skin ageing or dipping which is what the marketing was designed to imply.

Worst of all are those new instant over the counter "puffers" that do go through the skin's defences and pump up the skin, beyond its natural capabilities. The packaging claims that the results can mimic or replace injections. I fail to see how for more than a few hours. Without constant use, like injectables the artificially pumped up extra skin later relaxes back and is worse than before.

Some of these cosmeceuticals are not only sold under many of the leading French designer cosmetic labels but also, the same products are available in the physician's offices, which is disturbing. To fully understand how they all work you need to be a chemist and I am not, anymore than most physicians are, hence asking for proof. Once again, I repeat that I am even more sceptical about any over the counter cream that makes outlandish claims that are unsupported by human skin clinical trials.

Human growth factors (HGF)
They are another major focus for anti-ageing research by most big skincare companies. HGF can be applied topically and supposedly can have a big impact on skin repair and collagen production. Growth factors are large molecules, making them difficult for skin to absorb.

Although the efficacy of HGF has been substantiated in-vitro, it still lacks the backing of a large clinical study. Research into human growth factors is very complicated and intriguing, especially its long-term risk or stability when they are used in cosmetics and applied to skin every day. Research has examined HGF's effect in-vitro and one can watch the growth process of cells in a short period of time. But if excess HGF is added, the skin cells die sooner than they would have if no HGF were added.

HGH administration is considered controversial and it should not be used simply to improve aged skin. Until long-term safety/efficacy studies are completed, its topical use in cosmetics should be of concern to both consumers and dermatologists until more data is available on products containing human growth factors.

Having been so negative about most cosmeceuticals creams I should write something more about the ingredients found in some of other creams. I would recommend that you visit a highly reputable dermatologist before using any

- **Vitamen A creams** *Tretinoin (Retin-A)* and other acids, *Alpha Hydroxy Acids (AHA's), Glycolic acids, Polyhydroxy Acids (PHA's), Beta Hydroxy Acids* .
  Are all fundamentally for exfoliation/peeling.
- **Hydroquinone** and (less effective) *kojic acid, Alpha Arbutin* (is safer).
  Whitening/bleaching agents are for the reduction of brown pigment.
- **Vit E**
  Makes a sunscreen more effective, is an anti oxidant moisturiser, and prevent scars. It doesn't have to be topical, eat more Vit E, it comes to the surface where it neutralised free radicals in the cells and moisturises the skin.
- **Vitamin C**
  Is the only topical ingredient **I would recommend.**
  A deficiency is called scurvy, where the *collagen* cannot be produced and the skin breaks down. Vitamin C applied topically can boost the skin's vitamin C concentration by twenty fold. This is backed by strong scientific evidence.

Knowing this about vitamin C, I tried some recently, which was organic and sounded good. Without name/brand dropping, it was packaged in plastic orange coloured bottle, it smelt great and when applied, felt great, it was absorbent but later it irritated my eyes. Worse still, I woke up to find shopping bags under my eyes; maybe it is just a question of getting used to it? Maybe I have very sensitive skin? Maybe it was the brand?

However, just a couple of days later I read this: "Potentially, vitamin C can benefit the skin in two important ways. Firstly, vitamin C is essential for the synthesis of *collagen,* a key structural protein of the skin. Adding vitamin C to a culture of skin cells *(fibroblasts)* dramatically increases the synthesis of *collagen.* Secondly, vitamin C is an *antioxidant* and can help reduce skin damage caused by *free radicals*". So, when vitamin C is properly delivered into skin cells, there is a good chance to reduce wrinkles and improve skin texture.

Researching further, I discovered that unfortunately, there are some complicating circumstances that often disregarded by cosmetic manufacturers. First, vitamin C is relatively unstable (unless it is in a dry form). In the presence of air or other oxidising agents, vitamin C is easily converted to oxidised forms. The oxidised vitamin C is not only incapable of boosting collagen synthesis or scavenging free radicals but may actually promote free radical formation causing damage to vital molecules such as proteins and DNA. In poorly prepared or poorly stored skin care products, vitamin C may already be oxidised by the time you apply it to your skin. Second, only highly concentrated preparations (10% or more) deliver enough vitamin C to the cells to be topically effective.

Ah, now I know! The article goes on to say make your own and even then only 50% respond well. So where does that leave us, still in the dark? Not really, it just tells us that what our mothers told us was right; the old fashioned ideas of eating right, drinking plenty of water, sleep enough, staying out of the sun, away from alcohol and drugs are all the best prescription for healthy skin. More recently everyone agrees that we should add exercise to the equation. I and many doctors would remind you that exercising your face is no less important than exercising your body for a healthy, toned appearance.

Improvements in skin care creams are being made and I am currently researching all the latest creams in the hopes of finding something, which not only I could use, but perhaps could be marketed under a new **Fitface** label? Currently I rely on good old E45, a very simple dermatological over the counter moisturising lotion that soothes, softens and relieves dry and sensitive skin. It is perfume free – hypoallergenic. Although as a friend pointed out it is white and nothing in nature is white, therefore how good really is it? It just seems to work for me. The problem is that it is not FDA approved, although it is probably the cheapest, most widely used, everyday ("bog standard") moisturising lotion in the UK! Hence my search for its replacement, as Mummie gets fed up with sending it to me.

Alpha Lipoic acid
I have also been reading about the benefits of natural nontoxic *alpha lipoic acid.* Theoretically it is a very powerful antioxidant, anti-inflammatory agent, and can remove certain toxins. It can only be found in very small quantities in food. It is soluble in both fat and water. Apparently it works to improve the overall appearance of the skin. It is best in treating:

- Acne scars
- Sallow or dull skin
- Lines and wrinkles
- Under-eye bags and puffiness
- Enlarged pores

It is widely available in creams, lotions and masks from a range and variety of dermatologists and plastic surgeons and in some lines in limited distribution in department stores. I just don't know, most reports are good, but one was not and suggested it was overrated and substantiated studies on human skin were needed.

DMAE (dimethylaminoethanol)
Like all systems in the body, the nervous system ages and the amount of *acetylcholine* produced, as well as the effect of the chemical on the muscle is diminished. I have read that DMAE mixed in a cocktail with other nutrients, combined with an antioxidant base and applied topically can quickly and dramatically improve the appearance of sagging skin by helping cells to expel waste and hold on to valuable nutrients. DMAE won't accomplish anything approaching a well-performed surgical face-lift, but it is not useless either. In fact, DMAE may be the first agent proven in a study to have at least some positive effect on facial sag.

DMAE is a naturally occurring substance that facilitates the synthesis of a neurotransmitter acetylcholine. The mechanism of how DMAE firms the skin remains unclear; therefore, I will not include them here.

DMAE both internally and externally will result in better general health and an optimal nutritional environment for the skin. Additionally DMAE capsules have been found to help people increase cognitive function. But DMAE's best source is fish. I have yet to try it as being a vegetarian I don't eat fish, but the information sounds good. I looked for it in Public's (USA supermarket chain) but couldn't find it. I am off to Nutrition Smart (a health store near where I am currently living in West Palm Beach, Florida). But it will be too late in this edition for me to publish my findings.

I must admit that since menopause my skin has become much dryer, I drink more too, unfortunately meaning alcohol! Yes, I know, I know I should follow my own advice and drink much less; it is full of sugar, the collagen killer! Therefore, more than ever I need a richer moisturiser, so I am definitely on the hunt for something soft, natural, non allergic that actually is non greasy that will penetrate the skin. When I find it, I will, (of course) definitely share my knowledge with you.

In the mean/after time, (like you) I WOULD LOVE TO FIND A TOPICAL CREAM - that could make me look 10 years younger! Hey brilliant, no effort. Do, please write and tell me if you find one! I would love to know.

Natural spring water sprays

Are marketed to refresh your face with oxygenated water which they do, up to a point, but a plant or small spray with tap water does the same!

If nothing else sinks in *please give your money to a charity* rather than buy this product. There is no scientific proof whatsoever that this really is any better for the skin than tap water! Do not waste your money and I will not waste your time going into the details here. However, the one concern with tap water is the amount of chemicals in it, especially chlorine, which not only dries the but also, has toxicity issues for sensitive people. The chlorine is gassified when spayed and (need I mention Bhopal to remind you of the health dangers of chlorine gas in the extreme)?

I think normal tap water in a spray bottle to hydrate the face is excellent, I used one almost daily. Just ordinary tap water, in a plastic spray bottle container, applied whenever I feel like it. So refreshing; especially in Florida! Great too on an aeroplane just remember to take on board a very small spray bottle, empty at first and fill on board. Then I use a perfume container to put the water in, fabulously refreshing. A friend gave me a small bottle of real rose water in a handbag sized spray. The label says it is from a range of all natural products. So far I am impressed, not only does it smell divine but it also makes me feel special and it seems so much softer than my tap water. Watch this space or rather my blog!

Super facials

These are the latest anti-ageing techniques/ideas that are on the market to cash in on the late 2010 economic climate whereby face-lifts and Botox are becoming passé. Names vary, here are some popular ones:

> **The Buccal technique**
> An innovative intense facial massage; done from inside the mouth ("buccal" from the Latin for cheeks) to tackle the parts of the facial

musculature where tension and stress are stored. Therefore, for me, it is muscle building/manipulation done for you.

Simontherapie Collagen Restructuring Masque - the Parisian peel
A concoction of fruit acid is painted onto the skin before a warm electronically powered mask in placed on the face to remove dead cells. The treatment ends with a soothing cold cream mask to ease any redness that may be caused.

Fusion 3D Lift - the triple action facial
A highly sophisticated machine combines micro-dermabrasion acoustic wave therapy and infrared laser in one treatment.

CACI Ultimate - the 60-Minute face-lift
Dead cells are polished away with a disposable-tipped micro-dermabrasion tool. Then, blue and red LE light therapy works to destroy bacteria. Next, two hand-held probes are used to stimulate slack muscles to cause them to tighten.

The Super Charged Facial – the skin matters laser facial
Various techniques including IPL (intense pulsed light) and laser are incorporated to treat a plethora of skin concerns from sun damage to thread veins.

Homeo dermal facial
Holistic meets high-tech for those who prefer chemical-free remedies. The treatment combines micro-current technology with homeopathic products to improve skin quality and address health concerns by triggering the body's natural healing system.

Injectables and fillers

Are another quick fix alternative within the anti-ageing alternatives currently available. A series of injections are applied to the small facial muscles underlying visible lines on the face every three to six months, they temporarily paralyze the muscles, smoothing out the skin above. They appear to work almost instantly (although a week or so is recommended to see the full results) but at what cost, both in terms of pain, finance, risk and long term usage?

They are invasive as the needle penetrates the skin which generally causes swelling and bruising that should subside. As with all medical procedures complications are possible, they may include lumpiness (an uneven texture of the skin), an allergic reaction, infection, abscess or scarring. The possible side effects can take an age to disappear while others never completely vanish.

A friend of mine had her lips injected for months. However, now, that the *"trout pout"* has fortunately faded in popularity, sadly and she was left with a perpetually pulsating protruding pout that I suspect was from nerve damage.

Cosmetic fillers are not all alike and the same can be said for the technical skill of the person injecting the fillers. I am really appalled by the so called Botox parties where ladies get together, have a few glasses of wine and inject each other! More often than not, without a clue about what they are doing, without having the foggiest idea of where the muscles are; aided only by the bravado affect brought on by a few glasses of wine!

There are numerous different fillers on the market all claiming to be the best. They include a variety of materials, which last for different lengths of time and have different effects and uses. I cannot keep up with all the new miracle cures. It is a multibillion dollar industry and growing daily with the obsession for eternal youth and beauty. Having done so much research I find it all a little sad. However, I have included some of the most popular.

- **Botulinum toxin**

Botox is a drug made from a toxin produced by the bacterium Clostridium Botulinum which produces the deadliest toxin known to humans, 6 million times deadlier than rattlesnake venom! This same diluted toxin is injected into specific muscles to temporarily relax them, resulting in their inability to wrinkle the skin overlying the treated muscle. Botox injections work by weakening or paralyzing certain muscles or by blocking certain nerves. Botox is a poison and prolonged use causes the muscles to atrophy from lack of use.

It is only helpful for ***dynamic wrinkles*** (wrinkles in motion) and is not as effective on ***static wrinkles*** (wrinkles at rest) but prolonged use may help prevent those becoming dynamic wrinkles. It's not for me because I would be very concerned about the pain, expense of maintenance and the real possibility of it going lumpy. Worse still is that if you have artificially pumped up the skin and then can no longer afford the expense the stretch skin forms worse wrinkles. Therefore in the long term it actually exacerbates the situation, to rectify this - more Botox is required and the person becomes puffy looking with childlike chipmunk cheeks!

Where does the Botox go when it fails to work after 4/5 months? How does Botox dissipate inside our bodies? (Opinions differ):

> The toxin is a protein that prevents the release of a neuromuscular transmitter or the chemical from a nerve that goes to the muscle to tell it to contract. Because the nerve shuts down but continues to get signals from the brain that the muscle should work it sprouts new nerve endings. These don't have the Botox in them and as they hook up with the muscle the muscle regains function.
> **Christopher L. Hess, MD** - Fairfax Plastic Surgeon.
>
> Dr. Chen has provided a concise review. I would also add that in addition to travelling through the bloodstream, a recent animal study showed that Botox can travel backwards through the nerve to the Central Nervous System. The effect and consequences of this were unknown.
> **Otto Joseph Placik, MD** - Chicago Plastic Surgeon

- **Dermal fillers**

These are injectable substances which are used to restore or enhance fullness to the lips or to correct moderate to severe facial wrinkles and folds, such as nasolabial folds. Obviously your expressions change, however it is marketed as the easy way out for temporary results once again, of course, it involves risk even in the short term. The long term use is even more uncertain but definitely involves more pain, upkeep and cost.

There are many brand names, which I feel I should not list and therefore by virtual of inclusion subconsciously endorse.

Furthermore, I should add that the upper part of the face contains distinct groups of muscles that can be selected and paralyzed by a knowledgeable injector. However, in the lower part of the face, the muscle groups are less distinct making it far more difficult to inject these muscles accurately even by the most experienced professional. Let alone an inexperienced, newly trained practitioner who has perhaps just graduated from a "Hyaluronic Dermal Infusion Day" at the local college!

- **Natural fillers**

There is nothing natural about "fillers". However I suppose if you are going to have a needle stuck in your face, then I would assume that a "natural" product should be safer than a synthetic one. Although natural can be taken as euphemism the very thought of either idea, sounds simply ghastly.

Collagen type injections replenish the skin's natural collagen. The natural beauty of the skin is enhanced as the contour of the support structure is restored. These Bovine derived collagen products replace the collagen that your skin loses over time and are injected just beneath the skin, in the *dermis* where the body readily accepts it as its own.

There are bioengineered human collagen products that are used for similar but have the advantage of not requiring a skin test prior to the first treatment.

Autologen is an injection of your own collagen, extracted from another place on your body. There's no risk of allergic reaction, however, the results are only temporary. This may be good for people who aren't ready to commit to a permanent result.

Dermalogen is collagen extracted from deceased human donors. It's also called injectable Human Tissue Matrix. This is also a temporary fix, but your body should not reject it.

Collagen (as with all fillers) should be injected into your skin only by a trained health care professional. Please be careful and ask for proof of credentials/professional certification if you ignore my advice and resort to this type of treatment.

Fat from your own thighs or abdomen can also be injected. There's no risk of allergic reaction and you may achieve permanent results. This can also be implanted surgically.

However, injected fat may not last as long as some other materials. The fat is slowly absorbed by the body, although the amount of absorption is variable, and frequently hard to predict. Typically, more than half of the fat used in injectable treatments is absorbed with six months of the operation. Almost all patients will permanently retain some of the injected fat.

Fat is the first choice of material when injections are needed in deeper layers of tissue or larger volumes (greater than 10 cc).

A fat-injection procedure is a two-step process that may require more than one visit to the doctor. The fat must be harvested from somewhere on your own body, typically from the abdomen or hips. After it is extracted, it is placed in a centrifuge to separate the fat from surrounding tissues. The fat is then packed into a large syringe to accommodate its granular nature.

Because fat is a bit larger than other injectable materials, it is almost always injected more deeply into the skin. Volumes of up to 50 -100 cc can be used to cover the entire face. (Fat is the only injectable material that can be used at these larger volumes).

The side effects are swelling and bruising that lasts from days to several weeks unless there are complications from infection or anaesthetics.

HylaForm is a material created from natural body substances. There's no risk of infection, but you will need repeated treatments to maintain the result as it's only a temporary fix.

Stem cells fillers/face-lifts work by liposuctioning fat from the patient's own body and separating out the stem cells. They are then injected into the cheeks and frown lines. This procedure is done because stem cells replicate thereby rejuvenating the older facial tissue. This is often done in combination with a traditional face-lift but it can also be injected without performing surgery. It is a very, very expensive course of action.

Resurfacing techniques

Skin resurfacing using chemical peel, laser peel (see lasers) or **dermabrasion** or the gentler variation **microdermabrasion** skin-freshening technique.

Chemicals are placed on top of the skin to peel off the top layer. Microdermabrasion is a general term for the application of tiny rough grains to buff away the surface layer of skin. Many different products and treatments use this method, including medical procedures, salon treatments and creams and scrubs that you apply yourself at home.

Peels are generally mildly to extremely uncomfortable and can be very painful as the acid dissolves the skin. They almost always cause severe soreness and redness which should disappear within time and occasionally blistering. I am not a fan of subjecting the skin to such abuse. It can actually worsen conditions such as superficial red spider veins. They are costly and very abrasive. There can also be reactions and sometimes they peel off more layers than was intended. The results do not last. A friend of mine had one and a year later you would never have known.

The skin is designed to naturally shed without putting acid on your face! The top layer is dead skin which sloughs off naturally between 28 – 30 days in your twenties to 45 – 50 days in your sixties.

If you have had seriously bad acne scars, have brown spots or your skin is really damaged then the use of dermabrasion's and the results achieved are all relative.

Spa treatments

The *non invasive* spa treatments cannot really be compared as an alternative to hands free facial toning. The normal procedures on offer are not designed to tone muscles. They are all about the body beautiful and the feel good factor. All spas vary in terms of cost and range of specialist treatments.

Original spas were all about taking the waters, such as at Bath in southern England, the baths of Rome and Turkish baths. In the last fifty years the meaning has been transformed into meaning places of pure relaxation, natural beauty and healing within a calm and tranquil environment. Nowadays there are as many different types of treatments available as there are spas to go to, all claiming to have the answer to a more beautiful you. Anything goes from the traditional spas to the beauty shop in the mall offering laser and injectable solutions.

Treatments generally fall into two categories:

- **Non-invasive -** dealing with skin care, massages, body treatments, wraps, hydra facilities, waxing hair removal, eyebrow tinting, exfoliation, make up, manicures and pedicures.
- **Invasive -** which are a hybrid of day spa and medical spa, some of which are run under the supervision of a medical doctor. These offer such treatments as laser treatments, laser hair removal, IPL (intense pulsed light) treatments, microdermabrasion, photofacials, injectables (like Botox and fillers), chemical peels and skin tightening.
- A few offer even more specialised invasive laser treatments for Rosecea, pigmented lesions and thread veins.

Unfortunately because the very word "**spa**" does conjures up thoughts of traditional, pure, healthy and natural, many unnatural procedures are carried out in spa's. This allows invasive procedures to sound "natural/safe/normal" legitimizing them. There is nothing natural about sticking needles in you!

Without going into too many specifics non-invasive "treatments" spas mainly exist to encourage pampering, relaxing and self absorbed beautifying indulgences, they do just that. Generally they are designed to make you *feel* better and *feel* special. If you think some of the more unusual, mystifying treatments will work and make you look more gorgeous than you already are, then they probably will, simply enjoy them, go for it.

If on the other hand, they are more invasive procedures such as extremely vigorous massages that are not for the faint hearted, chemical peels etc then check, check, check and investigate the procedures on offer. Remember they are in business to take your money and at the same time make you look and feel good, if they don't then forget it!

Collagen Induction Therapy (CIT) aka Collagenesis (although I am unable to verify this term medically)

Also called **"skin needling"** is a procedure that involves puncturing the skin multiple times with fine needles to induce new collagen production and improve skin texture. The needles cause thousands of microscopic 'controlled injuries' to the deeper layers of the skin (the dermis) without tearing the skin. This induces the skin to begin a process of wound healing that is followed by the production of new collagen and elastin. The production of new collagen continues for up to 12 months after the procedure.

Lasers treatments

Currently there appear to be two main types of laser treatments on the market;
- one concentrates on resurfacing the superficial facial skin
- the other type purports to penetrate the underlying layers

I do not consider superficial laser treatments as an alternative to facial toning exercises. It is my understanding that they were designed for skin conditions such as; birthmarks, pigment or red blemish removal, mole removal, facial red veins and laser skin resurfacing, etc. They do seem to profess amazing results and **Fitface toning** alone will not reduce the appearance of already incurred fine red veins, sun spots or other pigments. However, please use caution when considering any of these treatments.

I suffer mildly from *Rosecea* and/or visible fine red veins, probably due to too much alcohol consumption. About 6 years ago, I decided to do something about it and sought the advice of my physician concerning what possible remedies were currently available and he recommended a series of laser treatments. He further suggested a practitioner, a nurse, whose laser experience extended to having been employed as the senior training nurse for a national group of laser treatments centres throughout the United Kingdom. So much for that!

Unfortunately, I was personally very disappointed with the results of the first treatment and never completed the course. I actually thought that I came out looking worse than when I went in. At the practise, immediately following the procedure, I looked quite red in the face. Later that evening, the colour worsened and during the night it progressed into my looking and feeling as if I had sunburn. By the morning it had manifested into the harsh reality that I had developed severe sunburn. I had begun to blister and immediately called the nurse for remedies. I was told to let my face scab and not to scratch, which I did and was reassured that I would soon look fine. I waited, as instructed, but as time passed I did not look fine, although admittedly it had settled down somewhat and was no longer sore and bright red. I felt so stupid at having been so gullible; enough to have thought it would work.

I let a few months pass and with little improvement I then complained. Although I had signed the disclaimer, I felt protected, as initially photos had been taken. The nurse was happy to discuss things and said that indeed I did look better and she would prove it by taking more photos and compare the two sets side by side. However, she was not always available and more time passed. Eventually, she took the photographs, had them developed and later still invited me in to review the two sets. The initial set clearly showed the veins and Rosecea on my face. However, in the later set I almost looked as green as the Incredible Hulk which proved her point that the redness had gone. She would not listen to my reasoning that the first set had a red tint to the photographs whereas the second had a green tint, and that they were completely different. She insisted she had done nothing wrong.

A year passed and my skin had healed. I wanted to travel for a year or two and to be honest I was too lazy to take the matter further. The veins and the redness were and are still there. I would like to try something again to remove them, if anyone can advise me of a safe, pain free treatment for Rosecea I would be happy to listen. From my experience, I would obviously advise extreme caution.

The marketing of these newest, latest types of lasers is that they heat the underlying structures of the skin and thereby promote collagen renewal and tone muscles. But I am not persuaded that they work or that they can just heat the underlying layers without damaging the upper skin tissues. I am also concerned about the short and long term side effects. Surely, these lasers must work in a similar way to the above lasers but at a lower frequency. I honestly don't know if they work and after my last disastrous experience I am too afraid to try.

They all make different claims and most claim to improve skin tone and rebuild collagen. They say heat is applied to shorten *collagen fibres* restoring some elasticity to the skin but what does this mean? *Is the fibroblast-stimulating* ingredient simply heat and the cells think they have been burnt? I think or rather know that is so. *Surely lasers just heat the skin?* Yes, to different temperatures which penetrate different layers? Are they not just to damage skin cells at different levels? How can this tone the skin, build collagen, elastin and strengthen muscle? Yes, they can burn down, to slowly destroy collagen and elastin, and yes, it will rebuild naturally. Is that how they rejuvenate, by stimulating collagen production? Is that not how the exercise works, by the breakdown and subsequent rebuilding of collagen? Yes. However when a doctor, uses different words to express the same thing for lasers it sounds sooooooo much better!

A doctor wrote this:

Laser treatments do stimulate the production of collagen in the dermal layer of the skin. It is actually the thermal (heat) injury induced by the lasers which stimulates the production of collagen in the dermal layer. I prefer to use fractional CO_2 lasers as they combine safety and efficacy. The fractional technology minimises the risk of pigmentation issues and scarring while still providing enough heat to stimulate collagenesis (production of collagen). Another treatment can also stimulate the production of collagen in the dermis without damaging the superficial skin (epidermis).

He goes on to names brands!

The radio frequency energy is transferred through the skin without damaging the superficial layers; it heats the deep dermis and thus stimulates the production of collagen.

I cannot keep up with all the new brand and product names but essentially lasers all work on the same principal as **Fitface** hands free toning, to breakdown collagen and elastin and let **nature rebuild** it. The only problem is that lasers do not also build muscles. They may be quicker but they are more painful, more risky and definitely more costly. Furthermore by such invasive methods to trick the fibroblasts into thinking they have been harmed by the sun doesn't this send the free radicals crazy, searching for their other electron? Perhaps I am just willing to be old fashioned and put in the effort required to exercise!

Okay, I am being negative, maybe lasers are just a quick fix, and certainly they work for some superficial skin resurfacing. Perhaps I just take pride in working for something, accomplishing something that is all me, not artificial. It doesn't matter perhaps to the world, maybe only me? I like me, and want to be me.

I would like to hear from anyone, with firsthand knowledge of laser treatments, whether positive or negative as far as toning the skin.

Devices

There are many different devices on the market but generally they fall into three categories:

1. Electrical muscle stimulation machines.
2. Mechanical gismos.
3. Face mask exercises.

The electrical muscle stimulation machines have been around for many years. They work by sending a mild electric current to the facial muscle which stimulates it into a contraction and then without any stimulus the muscle releases and so on. Whilst I have tried them, I do not think they are harmful, however I really did not see any results and it felt weird. Furthermore, by the time you set up the system and attach all the electrodes you might just as well have some fun doing a **Fitface toning** routine. For me they are a little like the body exercise machines, by the time you have set it all up you may as well have got on the floor and done 20 sit ups!

However, it does irritate me that one of the latest electronic gismo is being advertised by a celebrity who has publically admitted to having had not one but two face-lifts! One of which was famously a hugely expensive stem cell face-lift! She is also a regular promoter of growth hormone (see later) which supposedly stimulates growth, reproduction and regeneration. So I fail to be impressed by the so called results. Sadly, the manufacturers (via the advertisers) "dumb down the gullibility of the America audience" who unfortunately fall into the trap and fall prey to celebrity endorsements thereby believing such utter rubbish, purchasing the product. Personally I feel celebrities should be more ethical but then if L'Oreal/Channel etc approached me with a recurring multi-million contract would I refuse? Such is life.

The gadgets and gismos that I have come across normally only seem to target the mouth area and although I feel they may be of benefit to that specific area albeit that they are not reaching other important muscles that also need to be toned.

One of the latest more worrying devices is the face exercise mask. Fortunately the *Face Trainer*™ is marketed by No, No from Japan which says it all. This tight fitting facial mask is supposed to help you perform facial resistance-training exercises. In my opinion like the hands on facial exercises it can pull the skin beyond its normal limits thus causing wrinkles.

Last but not least is the Nintendo's Otona No DS Kao Natural Face-lift Training from Japan, which is a nifty little fun gadget but unfortunately I think, from some of the advertising I have seen it does not only have hands free exercises, which as you know is why I think **Fitface** is hands down the best of all facial exercise regimes to follow.

Growth hormone (GH)

A protein-based polypeptide hormone that *stimulates growth*, reproduction and regeneration in humans and other animals, but can they in the face?

Claims for **GH** as an anti-ageing treatment date back to 1990 when the *New England Journal of Medicine* published a study wherein **GH** was used to treat 12 men over 60. At the conclusion of the study, all the men showed statistically significant increases in lean body mass and bone mineral, while the control group did not. The authors of the study noted that these improvements were the opposite of the changes that would normally occur over a 10 to 20 year ageing period. Despite the fact the authors at no time claimed that GH had reversed the ageing process itself, **their results were misinterpreted** as indicating that **GH** is an effective anti-ageing agent.

A Stanford University School of Medicine survey of clinical studies on the subject published in early 2007 showed that the application of **GH** on healthy elderly patients increased muscle by about 2 kg and decreased body fat by the same amount. However, these were the only positive effects from taking **GH.** No other critical factors were affected, such as bone density, cholesterol levels, lipid measurements, maximal oxygen consumption, or any other factor that would indicate increased fitness. Researchers also did not discover any gain in muscle strength, which led them to believe that **GH** merely let the body store more water in the muscles rather than increase muscle growth. This would explain the increase in lean body mass.

Hormone replacement therapy (HRT) or aka (in Britain) **Hormone therapy (HT)**

That is a system of medical treatment for surgically menopausal, *perimenopausal* and to a lesser extent, postmenopausal women. It is based on the idea that the treatment may prevent discomfort caused by diminished naturally circulating estrogen and progesterone hormones. It involves the use of one or more of a group of medications designed to artificially boost hormone levels. The main types of hormones involved are estrogens, progesterone or progestins, sometimes testosterone. It is often referred to as "treatment" rather than therapy.

I had terrible menopausal symptoms 24/7 hot flushes and night sweats, no not perspiration, more like swimming the English Channel in bed all night. It drove me crazy getting up, showering, drying off, and making the bed - only for it to happen a few hours later. The only time it stopped was when I slept with my boyfriend, weird, I put it down to creating the right sex hormones, who knows? I sympathise with anyone suffering menopausal symptoms and I was the first one down to see my doctor when none of the herbal type remedies worked. Bring on those drugs!!

Had I been in American at that time I may well have tried *Biodenticals*, the marketing all sounds better, "natural" but sadly my research has done nothing to convince me that they are better.

Bioidenticals

Hormone therapy can increase a woman's risk of heart attacks, strokes, blood clots and cancer. And despite some celebrities claims that non FDA approved bioidenticals are "natural" and safer, they are actually synthetic, just like conventional hormones and FDA approved *bioidenticals* from pharmacies - and there are no conclusive clinical studies showing that they are less risky. That's why endocrinologists advise that women should take the smallest dose that alleviates symptoms, and use them only as long as they're needed.

Weird and wacky

And I thought colonic irrigation was crazy!

IV Drip

The latest trend in the USA in order to restrict ageing is an IV drip, a vitamin cocktail. You get hooked up to a machine for 20 minutes. Relax, knowing that the nutrients are being injected directly into your bloodstream, it is already popular in Japan and is now gaining popularity in USA to fight against ageing. Ageing causes changes in the digestion and absorption of nutrients. Many physical changes occur along the digestive tract itself. The theory is that by injecting a vitamin cocktail mix directly into the veins it will give you quick results by boosting the energy which gives a glow to the skin. Caution should be exercised here, my research suggests that "yes", while this may have some merit for very elderly patients there is no merit for younger persons as "**digestion**" is very complex and potentially injections could be disruptive, or at the very least alter the natural body processes.

Even in the elderly, imagine giving a 10oz steak to an elderly relative, they would be up all night!

IV Chelation therapy

Is used, albeit differently, by both allopathic (conventional Western) medicine and alternative medicine as a means of purging toxic metals and minerals from the body. Practitioners of chelation therapy argue that it is an effective way of removing toxins and harmful body wastes, as well as helping to prevent or treat atherosclerosis, heart attacks, strokes, and circulation problems.

The most popular form of chelation therapy practised by alternative practitioners employs a drug called EDTA (ethylene diamine tetraacetic acid) administered intravenously. EDTA is approved by the Food and Drug Administration (FDA) for treatment of lead and heavy metal poisoning but not for other forms of toxicity or circulatory problems. EDTA works by attaching itself to specific minerals, which are carried out of the body via urinary excretion.

An intravenous solution of vitamins, minerals, and the chelator (substance that binds particular ions) EDTA is prepared. EDTA is a substance known for its ability to pull heavy metals out of the body. This is infused into the bloodstream through a vein.

EDTA leaves the body in the same form by which it entered, but on its way out, it chelates metals and minerals from the body. Patients usually undergo between 10 and 20 *chelation* treatments over a period of weeks or months. Each treatment lasts several hours, during which patients can read or watch a movie.

Leeches

Just when I thought that enough was enough! Demi Moore speaks to David Letterman, a popular USA TV host, about leeches in March 2008. Apparently, while they are biting down on you, engorging them, getting fatter and fatter, swelling with your blood, until they flop off punch drunk fashion, they are actually simultaneously detoxifying your blood by releasing an enzyme into the blood stream. Generally you bleed for quite a bit and the treatment is uncomfortable according to the actress but a little Lamaze breathing helps her get past the pain! If Demi believes that leeches are the way to detoxify then it must be, mustn't it? After all she is beautiful and married to a stud! Whatever! What's next? I can only hope that it was only a publicity stunt to sell her latest film, however where she goes, so the fans will follow. Recent royalty has believed in colonic irrigation! So who am I to poke fun? Thank goodness that craze has passed.

Although it sounds bizarre, leeches do have a place in modern medicine. In 2004, the Food and Drug Administration (FDA) cleared the commercial marketing of leeches for medicinal purposes for the first time when it granted approval to Ricarimpex SAS a French company.

According to the FDA, leeches can help heal skin grafts by removing blood pooled under the graft and restore blood circulation in blocked veins by removing pooled blood. Leeches have been used as an alternative treatment to blood-letting and amputation for several thousand years. They reached their height of medicinal use in the mid 1800's. Today they are used in medicine throughout the world as tools in skin grafts and reattachment surgery. Fine for medical purposes but for cosmetic enhancement, really!!!!

Skull lifts

I kid you not! Yes skull lifts may come as the next generation of anti-ageing cosmetic surgical procedures, designed for those who must have the latest treatment. Apparently the bones of the face move with age and contribute to the ageing look of our faces, it's not just our skin that goes south with age! However research is focused on injections to prevent the bone shift rather than using a knife to correct it.

A very personal story

Over the years I have read and researched much about facial exercises, facial surgery and injections and as I wrote in the introduction of **Fitface - the natural face-lift** my catalyst for beginning facial exercises was witnessing first hand an early face-lift which was more akin to butchery. However, time has moved on, there have been many medical advances in face-lift techniques as well as my personal experience of them.

I now owe my daughter's life to the skill of a team of British plastic surgeons who put her face back together following a horrific accident. She had been smashed face first onto a brick wall by a cargo truck whilst walking through Kingston-upon-Thames High Street, England one Saturday morning in the spring of 2003. She had been following her father to get to her parked car; he took a short cut, walking between a wall and a parked truck. The driver turned on his engine, went into first gear, moved forward, she screamed…

The emergency services went into action; they craned cars out of the parking lot (car park), landed the helicopter and gave her emergency medical treatment. I was later told she was still impaled and conscious when they arrived and she would not release her cell (mobile) phone as she was trying to talk, saying "Call Mummie", before they knocked her out. I was also told that a lady had opened a brand new blanket that she had just bought and threw it on top of my daughter to stop her from going into shock. They stabilised her, put her on life support machines and then transported her by helicopter to the Royal London hospital which specialises in facial trauma, oral and maxilla facial surgery. She was only just 18.

Somehow, through the shock and a haze of streaming tears, I made it to London in about 2 hours aided by a couple of old Vaillum that I had found. I arrived and ran through emergency entrance and in my state asked an ambulance driver where my little girl, he something like she didn't make it. I hurled into the hospital and somehow found reception and found that she was clinging to life in the trauma ward. I was taken to a special waiting room but was in no mood to make small talk with her father. I waited in the general emergency room. After waiting about a further hour or so, I was told I could see her. Brittany's father and I were taken to the trauma ward.

I first saw her in a body brace, like a fibreglass open casket with metal bars across the front opening; one was on her forehead holding her rigidly still. They had stabilised her life support systems. She looked horrific; with her right eye hanging out, with all sorts of tubes in her mouth, vomiting blood and guts out from the sides of them. Machines were buzzing and throbbing everywhere.

The next time I saw her was that evening after she had been transferred to the intensive care. The medical staff had prepared her for a frontal lope by shaving off a 2 inch wide section of her hair across the top of her head from ear to ear. I now think it was as a precaution for a possible emergency brain surgery but fortunately at the time, I thought it was for major reconstructive surgery to rebuild her face. Her whole face was squashed and had been swollen into the shape of a rugby ball (like an American football). She was featureless, with her lovely long blonde locks of hair, of which she was so proud, matted with blood. I just sobbed uncontrollably.

The male nurse was terrific, he talked to her as if she was conscious, calling her by name, treating her as if she was human, not just a pile of lifeless flesh. He attended to her dressings, taped her right eye back over and told me cheerily that he thought she had been extraordinarily lucky and that she would only loose an eye! I was horrified and thought that she would rather be dead.

Sometime later, when she regained consciousness they asked her to move her finger, I choked back the tears, trying to look strong, seeing that she was able to and wiggle her toes, she would not be a paraplegic a feeling of utter relief gushed over my entire body, I was euphoric. They were then able to conduct a brain scan and found that she was remarkably physically uninjured except for 21 fractures in her face. She had no visible signs of brain injury; she would not be a vegetable. They had asked her silly questions to which she was just able to whisper a one word plausible answer. I can't remember what it was, just my feelings of relief.

Earlier, I had contemplated pulling the plug and serving 30 years if the results of the scan were negative. However my original thoughts were distracted by trying to focus on keeping her alive by shouting "BREATHE" whenever the monitor line began to flat line, something she says she still remembers although unconscious!

The next morning her father and I had a consultation with the chief surgeon, he required recent photos as soon as possible. He explained the complexity of the operation sensitively but in graphic terms, detailing how they would pull the face off, cut around the eyes and leave only fine lines. Hysterical, I begged them not to cut her but to wait because I knew that at her age, she wouldn't want to live if she looked horrendous. The consultant insisted that it would only be minor scarring like the fine lines that surrounded my eyes, "Yes but I'm 47!" I retorted. Her father thought I had totally lost the plot but I pleaded with the surgeon, holding on to his suit lapels, "Imagine if it was your daughter!" Through the fuzz of memories I think he said he had a daughter slightly younger than mine. He said he would consult his colleagues and get back to us.

They agreed to wait until the swelling had gone down before making a final decision on the condition that they would operate immediately if her life was in danger. There was a new arrival in intensive care and as she was out of immediate danger she was moved to the critical ward. We constantly reassured her that she looked fine, that it wasn't too bad but every now and then it got too much for me and I retreated to wail in private. A few days later she was allowed visitors and got out of bed. Attached to her machines she looked like the "Exorcist", I do not exaggerate one of her girlfriends fainted at the very sight of her. She was very strong, she always had been, it was the way I had raised her to be secure and brave, I wanted her to be the opposite of me. Only occasionally did she let her guard down and show any anxiety about having surgery. I told her that the surgery was imperative. It was not optional. She had no choice; sign the consent forms; it was going to be done.

Incredibly nature took its course and rebuilt the severely damaged eye muscle connection and after <u>no mirrors</u> and "Nil by Mouth" for 5 days a team of surgeons operated on her through her mouth for six hours. Unbelievably they implanted five plates, 25 screws and a crown, rebuilt her nose from her ear cartilage and did all this without a single visible cut!

Within a week she was back at home. Within a month amazingly, her previously thought irreversibly damaged sensations of hot and cold returned, followed shortly by her sense of taste and smell. Within six weeks she jetted off to Greece on holiday with her final year classmates with the complete approval of her surgeon. If you had seen her then or now you would never ever have guessed that she had anything done to the face she was born with. Phenomenal!

Most remarkable of all her recovery was her bravery and total lack of emotional trauma, unlike me. I was and continue to be amazed at her attitude. She told me that it didn't hurt at the time when she was impaled and that her one overriding thought was that she was not going to die. Later it hurt but during her recovery she kept insisting that she would not allow the accident to ruin her life, she would not dwell on any traumatic issues and that was and is final. She told me that if anything, it made her feel stronger, really doing justice to the phrase "if it doesn't kill you it will make you stronger."

Perhaps it's true. She has certainly done more than most people her age, currently 25. She went on to obtain an honours degree in Languages and travelled the world with a back pack. She now lives with her partner in Australia, works in tourism and lives each day as she knows only too well how short life can be.

The reason why I am sharing this story with you is to show that **I am not at all opposed to cosmetic surgery in the right circumstances,** quite the contrary. I endorse their work when required, for there are some appalling medical or hereditary conditions, deformities, accidents and diseases which can only be corrected with surgery. I should also like to take this opportunity to extend my immense gratitude, admiration and appreciation to the team of plastic surgeons, Simon Holmes, Mr. Porn, the paramedics, ambulance crew, nurses and staff at the Royal London and St. Bart's Hospital in 2003. With a special mention to the London fire brigade and the Helicopter Emergency Medical Services who kept her alive initially and brought her safely through the major trauma to the hospital.

Medical professions definitions of surgeon's specialties

Definition of Oral and Maxillofacial surgeons
Specialise in the treatment of facial, mouth and jaw disorders such as cancer, facial and jaw joint pain and disfigurement and deformity. They are also trained in reconstructive and microsurgery, using other parts of their patient's bodies - such as hips and ribs - as well as titanium plates and screws to rebuild the face.

Definition of Plastic surgeon

A surgeon who specialises in reducing scarring or disfigurement that may occur as a result of accidents, birth defects, or treatment for diseases, such as melanoma. Many plastic surgeons also perform cosmetic surgery that is unrelated to medical conditions, such as rhinoplasty to change the shape of the nose.

Definition of Cosmetic Surgery

Cosmetic Surgery is a subspecialty of medicine and surgery that uniquely restricts itself to the enhancement of appearance through surgical and medical techniques. It is specifically concerned with maintaining normal appearance, restoring it, or enhancing it beyond the average level toward some aesthetic ideal.

Rhytidectomy

A face-lift. A surgical procedure designed to reduce the visible signs of ageing in the face.

Facial surgery vs. Facial exercises

Quite by chance, whilst browsing in a major book sellers in Florida I happened across a beautiful woman's glossy magazine, thumbed a couple of pages and thought I would enjoy reading it. At home and upon further inspection, it became clear that it had nothing to do with the normal beauty tips, articles and fashion ideas. Instead it was packed from cover to cover with cosmetic procedures of one kind or another whether performed by the knife or the needle. I was impressed by the fabulous pictures of all the stars, thought how wonderful they looked and how simple it all sounded until I woke up from my momentary absorption. Such is the power of the media to sway public opinion, even upon me (who is strongly anti cosmetic surgery for pure vanity) and none is greater than in the USA.

I live in Florida and I am constantly bombarded by advertisements offering one cosmetic surgical procedure or another either on the radio or TV; therefore it is perhaps not surprising that Florida has perhaps the greatest acceptance of cosmetic surgery in the world. Day in and day out the radio/TV and magazines all expound the virtues of surgery or injections at readily available discounts. Hardly ever does one hear from the other side, the disasters, but it is not far away. Look at my website or try searching Google with negative input like Botox gone wrong or a bad face-lift, it's not hard to find if you look.

The TV show in England (July 2010) is the Ugly Side of Beauty, a Channel 4 documentary, a new series in which Dr Christian Jessen warns of the risk of cosmetic surgery. Unbelievably he sets up a bogus discount practise in a British high street with two attractive young promotions girls without medical training or information. They simply sign up "wannabe's" on discount price alone. I am astounded, thinking perhaps there is no place for **Fitface** sense.

One of the major developments in the cosmetic surgery industry is that the goal posts of aesthetically perceived beauty by women have moved beyond reality. Whereas once, a person with a really ugly feature, for example an exceptional hooked bulbous nose had surgery, it is now performed legitimately on very pretty young TV presenters who rather than lack looks lack self esteem. I do sometimes wonder about the ethics of surgeons and am alarmed that women are being "surgically enhanced to the point of science fiction" as aptly described by a friend whilst people watching at an outside café in South Beach Miami.

What concerns me the most is that the acceptance level of cosmetic surgery now transcends into everyday life and that the age of girls desiring surgery grows ever younger, infiltrating their very impressionable minds. Most ladies of my age and older grew up dressing dolls. Life has not changed much except that it is now performed virtually (like many things) on a computer screen. The game is to design and dress the most beautiful woman in the world, options include diet pills, boob jobs and face-lifts! Worst still is that some mothers not only condone but actually support and may even encourage their teenage daughter's behaviour.

I read a novel last year in which a Manhattan socialite gave her daughter surgery for her 16th birthday. The child wanted to fit in with her friends at school. She had SUCH low self esteem, a lack of confidence and went along with her mother's idea of having surgery. She had a boob job; a new nose and a tummy tuck however she was blissfully unaware of her small sister who was looking on horrified and her distress caused by the pain she observed until after the fact. A month or so later she had made a full recovery and was delighted. The story continued to explain that her 10 year old sister later begged her mother for surgery. Whatever happened to being just okay within your own skin?

Yes, the above is just a game and the other a novel but the women who desire surgery are getting younger and younger and children are operated on with their parents consent. I feel certain that their opinions are formed not only by the media but also by the attitudes of their parents. My wealthy mature girlfriends in the USA are vehemently in favour of surgery despite the enormous risks and costs which to most of them is immaterial. Personally I feel a sad reflection of their self esteem however they assure me that it is to the contrary. They want to be the best they can be and are prepared to go to any lengths to get there. They see the option of facial surgery as empowering; something to make them strong. However, if these women, only just thought seriously about it, they would understand nothing could be further from the truth. Wouldn't they? "Our Bodies, Ourselves" was a feminist statement, for women to accept themselves as they are and to give up disguises to appeal to men. Have these women? I wonder what they would think about what my real research revealed.

Whilst conducting my investigations into facial cosmetic surgery I decided to interview men and ask their opinions, after all I surmised that any woman crazy enough to go through facial cosmetic surgery must want to attract the opposite sex (or keep what they already had, at home - interested); despite what they may say. The answers were not what I had been expecting especially from single men in the USA who were with or had been with women that had had surgery or invasive procedures performed. I consider needles invasive although they are advertised as non-invasive, the needle punctures the skin doesn't it and a foreign body is injected?

Far from being against the idea, the men were all for it, often paying for their girlfriends or wives to have surgery! Why? I was shocked. I thought men wanted naturally beautiful women. But "No", they answered honestly. They felt that any women who was prepared to go to those lengths of pain, money and suffering for their man or to be more attractive to men were the women who would be most likely to "Put out more" sexually to please their man or to keep their man happy.

I can only tell you what they told me, don't shoot the messenger! So, women may have equal pay in the workforce, but it would seem they are in reality more subservient than ever! So much for women's liberation! Perhaps it is as one man commented "a perverse form of the chastity belt!" Other men commented that they could be a fat ugly bastard but so long as they had money they could get whatever cute chick they wanted. No wonder wives feel insecure. Another standard response, often repeated – in so many words was, "You don't see us doing it, do you, unless a guy's gay or just plain stupid?"

I further explored this idea of gender inequality within the 21st Century's fashion of the self harm culture and found some quite disturbing evidence. Many in depth articles cited that socially approved self injury was a practise of violence against women enforced by social control for the creation of male dominance and female subordination. In Western society that oppression translates itself to self mutilation; destroying human tissue without suicidal intent, chosen and inflicted upon women by themselves, in order to be more appealing to men.

I leave you to draw your own conclusions or to read further, see the internet - **Shelia Jeffrey's** - is professor of Social and Political Sciences, University of Melbourne, Australia has some very interesting articles and books. She writes passionately about her views that the most common form of severe self-mutilation by proxy is cosmetic surgery; the practises in which women and some men, request others to cut up their bodies - as in cosmetic surgery, transsexual surgery, amputee identity disorder, pursuit of limb amputation and other **forms of sadomasochism - self-mutilation by proxy,** which overwhelmingly affects women. She notes that many of the forms of self harm are promoted to women by television shows and the advertisements of surgeons. It is powerful thought provoking reading not for the faint hearted.

Then of course, there is the other and lighter side of the coin. Men who were vehemently against the idea of a surgeon's knife or a needle getting anywhere near their wives, those men generally thought that their wives or girlfriends were perfect anyway, just the way they were. So there was no need. It was too preposterous for most of them to even consider logically; "Just plain silly!" Ah, how sweet. All (without) were very concerned with the practical medical risks and took the thought of any surgery, seriously. One man told me that he could not bear to lose his wife and would not want to live a day without her. Another man who's wife had died young of cancer said he would have then and would today, give all he had, as he was a multi-millionaire, just to spend one more day with her even now, even though she would now look much older. He chuckled and went on to say that it would be a bit funny if she hadn't aged because he had and that was how things were meant to be, to grow old together.

I posed the question of surgery to grandmothers and children. The grandmas were understandably generally against the idea of any surgery whatsoever with the exception of the rare glamorous granny in the USA. Obviously, most of young children thought it was nuts, ghastly. They understood the basics of cosmetic surgery and couldn't bear the thought of their Mummy's having any pain, the blood, yuk! They didn't want their mothers to change and loved them just the way they were. Early teens, most especially in Europe were adamantly against the idea, a group endorsing a remark made by one of them, "Until men have routine penis extensions why should I do anything!"

Some older teenage girls in the USA however offered some real insight. One girl said that many of her friends were considering changing themselves because they were not happy with the way they looked. "Why not be perfect?" Such is the peer pressure to conform even to abnormal behaviour.

Fortunately, not everyone sees the developments in cosmetic surgery as progress, Abigail Saguy; a professor of sociology at UCLA thinks that our growing obsession with surgery is unhealthy. "It's shocking that those women are so desperate not to age naturally," she says. "Is it really worth going to these extraordinary lengths just to feel acceptable?"

I investigated the physiological aspects of having facial surgery further and found more alarming information. This is not a medical journal and therefore I will keep this short. Basically, evidence showed that depressed people are more likely to have surgery than those who are not. Often they are looking to change the external to improve the internal. Self mutilation is a way of expressing pain and depression is anger turned inwards, therefore the link exists. For further readings see the internet. Interestingly, persons suffering with body dysmophic disorder have to persuade surgeons more voraciously to operate than the rest of us, which one could argue is the sole reason cosmetic surgery exists.

Doesn't anyone seriously consider the real extent of the risks - both mental, physical and more importantly the psychological effects of having a face-lift or facial surgery?

It is such a radical surgical procedure that face-lifts are performed under a general anesthetic! Here are some of the risks:

1. The possible complications that could arise from the anaesthetic alone are huge in addition to all the other possible unknowns like infections, allergic reactions, shock, **seroma,** (a pocket of clear serous fluid that sometimes develops in the body after surgery. When small blood vessels are ruptured, blood plasma can seep out; inflammation caused by dying injured cells also contributes to the fluid) pulmonary complications or even death can occur. Yes, it does happen and yes, it could be you!

2. The possibility of nerve damage ranges from mild numbness and twinges to strange sensations that are often felt post operatively. Some continue for years, or worst still result in severe nerve damage.

3. The probable or rather inevitable scarring, wherever it may be, if you cut the skin it naturally scars.

4. The thinning of stretched skin with the subsequent loss of elasticity can result in an opaque look, like a porcelain mannequin, does that look attractive?

5. Think about the psychological implications of considering changing yourself so alarmingly. "It doesn't look like me anymore!" The loss of ones identity and individuality encourages further procedures especially as the face age doesn't match the age of the body.

6. By having just one surgical procedure done it makes the other untouched "bits" of you look even older than they really are. To obtain a completely new look other procedures are required. A forehead, an eye and brow lift with possible cheek and chin implants! Maybe the next lift is to include the muscles too?

7. Personally, I feel the mental aspect of resorting to aesthetic cosmetic surgery to be the most alarming consequence. Western society is broadcasting and enforcing propaganda that I am not allowed to age gracefully and that I ought to resort to cutting myself, for me this is disturbing. Perhaps more disturbing is that I have to personally stand up and be counted as actually liking myself just the way I am!

8. The repeated procedures which are needed every 10 years at best and the addictiveness of surgery as opposed to the rewards become less and less satisfying. It can become a never ending treadmill. A lift does not arrest the ageing process.

9. The limited choice of procedures (on offer) to choose from creates the cookie cutter look. We all know the "Cat face", "Chinese look", the "death mask pull" the turned up "Bunny nose", the Trout pout", not to mention the greatest problem, the loss of face asymmetry.

10. As fashion changes, what was once great one day is out the next. Its bad enough trying to keep it together with clothes, it's quite another with your face!

11. There is a loss of emotions that are unable to be portrayed on a "lifted face." It is replaced with a blank uninspiring unrevealing clean canvas. Loss of expressions, loss of subtle communications - communication is 93% body language, facial expressions must account for most of that!

12. The pain and suffering endured by the patient is not to be looked upon too lightly unless you have an extraordinary pain threshold. It is not a pleasant business despite, what the brochures might say! Just be realistic, you are cut, you bleed, you are stitched back up, given pills, etc.

13. The real time of recovery and initial downtime caused by delayed healing is yet another issue that is so overlooked. Even simple procedures are not automatic. The body needs time to heal, it does not happen overnight.

In 2006, nearly 11 million cosmetic procedures were performed in the United States alone. Today (2010) the number of cosmetic procedures performed in the United States has increased over 50 percent since the start of the 21st century. Nearly 12 million cosmetic procedures were performed in 2007, with the five most common surgeries being breast augmentation, liposuction, nasal surgery, eyelid surgery and abdominoplasty. The increased use of cosmetic procedures crosses racial and ethnic lines in the U.S., with increases seen among African-Americans and Hispanic Americans as well as Caucasian Americans. In Europe, the second largest market for cosmetic procedures, cosmetic surgery is a $2.2 billion business. Cosmetic surgery is now very common in countries such as the United Kingdom, France, and Germany.

The message is clear that Americans are embracing cosmetic surgery and that these treatments are becoming more "main stream." With this large number of procedures across the country and the diverse group of doctors that perform them, the number of patients dying from surgery is an extremely small fraction of one percent. So how does an affluent and educated woman like Donda West, a retired professor and former chairwoman of the Chicago State University English department, die from plastic surgery? See the Internet.

What are the benefits of facial exercise?

They are listed more fully in an earlier in Chapter 3, however to reiterate the salient points.

Fitface is truly a non invasive, totally natural means of tightening the underlying muscles to firm the face, bringing back tone and improving the texture of the skin by increasing the blood supply carrying nutrients and taking away damaged cells. It is a slower, more natural, organic, preventative approach to anti-ageing.

The real question to ask yourself is, should you choose Fitface toning or surgery?

However, I think the question is too stupid to be taken seriously; of course the answer should be **Fitface toning. Facial exercise** is far superior to most aspects of aesthetic facial cosmetic surgery. My flippant response to my posing a stupid question can be put down to my British sense of humour. Besides it makes a grisly subject fun. I have left the answers to the Fitface debate unanswered. I believe you can answer them for yourself. It is the pain free, sensible alternative to ever needing a face-lift.

Fitface vs. surgery
The truthful consultation

Questions that you should ask a surgeon	Tongue in cheek - but honest responses/answers to genuine concerns that should be addressed by anyone considering facial surgery.
Is it pain free?	No, but you can have lots of really strong pain killers and take time off work to recover at home or be treated by a nurse at a convalescent nursing home.
Could I scar?	Yes, you definitely will, but we can hide them as best we are able. It all depends on how many areas you would like us to correct at once, how well the surgery goes and how well you heal naturally.
Are there any risks?	Yes of course, this is going to be major surgery under a general anaesthetic. All radical invasive surgery carries the risks of possible infections, complications or reactions, even death but that hardly ever happens.

Will any thing you do be irreversible?	No not if there were to be nerve damage or you really didn't like any radical results we achieved and we had cut off too much skin. This is because the more surgeries you have the less natural material we have to put things right. But don't worry, if you do look scary we will take some skin from somewhere else on your body and fix you up. We can even take cartilage from your ears or ribs! The cost of course will be down to you.
Can I have everything fixed at once?	Maybe. It all depends on what you want to have done. Firstly you must choose what type of lift; we have about 6 major ones to choose from plus many, many more minor lifts. Then you need to consider implants perhaps for the cheeks and chin, dental work and then what types of fillers etc plus anything else you want done to your neck, (another serious area to consider).
Will the texture of my skin improve?	No, not the actual skin itself it will get worse but you will look better because we stretch the skin which makes it look smoother initially but that makes it thinner and more see-thru.
Is it expensive?	Yes, but it does depend on which country you go to, to have an operation, who performs the surgeries, what bits you want to have done and when? We could start a payment plan and tackle the most serious parts first.
Will I look younger and fabulous?	I hope so, the first one is the best, if you don't look better you can always sue and I'll settle out of court because I can't afford the bad publicity, besides I have loads of insurance and you must sign a waiver before I proceed.
How long does it last?	Oh years, 5, 7 maybe even 10 if you are extremely lucky but then you can always see me again for another one, I'll be here for you to help make me richer.
Is it fun?	No! You wouldn't get me under the knife.

Doesn't anyone really care about the consequences of cosmetic surgery purely for vanity or to supposedly retard the natural ageing process? **Is it just me?** Surely things have gone too far? I am all for going to spas, looking good, taking care of yourself and even believe that looking better makes you feel better but there must be limits? Mustn't there? I guess not?

Okay, maybe it's just me that's weird. Maybe it's because I'm British? Maybe I am misguided, all wrong. Maybe the knife is the ONLY answer.

So let's forget about what **we all know** about diet, exercise and yes ageing - growing old! Maybe we should not exercise? Maybe we shouldn't even think about what we eat? Maybe ageing doesn't happen to everyone?

But no, seriously, it is common sense to eat nutritiously and exercise which includes exercising your face. I cannot promise you an instant change in your appearance, it will take time, dedication and effort but the results are more gracious, more flattering, showing the wonderful unique character of your face with results that grow with you.

I fought with my conscience about what to write with reference to all the women, who are like me, single and trying to keep up with the "in-crowd" and look great or as best one is able in ones mature single years. Are these women so wrong to consider having or having had surgery? What would I have done, should I not have followed the exercise toning route? It is difficult for me to say, I have done **Fitface** for years. So really it would be impossible for me to walk in their moccasins and answer. But then, I thought harder about the rest of my body. My breasts leave much to be desired, they are not those of my twenties. Would I have a "boob" job? The answer is most definitely "No". Why? Because until men routinely have an operation for droopy balls, not a pretty sight, I will not have an operation for droopy boobs, it's all too silly. As we all grow older, we should all learn, that with age comes wisdom, knowing there is more to a person than the superficial. Yes, easy to say but that is another book.

HOWEVER... perhaps you should forget what I have said and do what your heart tells you to do especially if your philosophy is "I want it now". You are not alone 14 million Americans chose cosmetic enhancing procedures last year alone. The power of advertising: creating a need and then filling it. I can't believe that anyone really wants surgery but if I was ill of course I would have an operation. My purpose here it to try to prevent a face-lift from ever being necessary; which obviously it is not, they are never necessary.

SUMMARY
- Take care of your face at every layer.
- No product or treatment can be effective at every level.
- All products and treatments affect different layers of the skin.
- Each product and treatment was designed specifically to penetrate to that level.

- Topical collagen or large molecule products do not work.
- Be wary of "puffers".
- Injectables have risks and need to be administered by an experienced professional.
- Facial surgery is surgery with all the associated risks.
- Face-lifts of today cut and tighten slack muscles. **Fitface** is all about toning facial muscles; surely prevention is better than cure?

The choice is yours.
There is an alternative

Fitface

Part 2

FACE EXERCISES

With photographs showing you how to exercise

Chapter 6

The Foundations

The Fitface Toning Rules

Essential reading!

<u>**Do not perform these exercises**</u> if you have ever had any facial surgery, have used any Botox, derma fillers or injectables without first consulting a dermatologist or surgeon (as applicable). **Fitface toning** exercises are preventative measures to avoid or postpone invasive procedures.

1. Do not perform **Fitface toning** exercises for at least 6 months if you have had a laser or chemical peel as your skin will be fragile. Consult with your dermatologist or plastic surgeon as to precisely how many weeks or months it will be until your skin is fully healed.
2. Do not exercise if you have sunburn, the skin will be tight and fragile. Wait until the natural oils and body's own hydration returns to your skin.
3. Do not exercise if you are on pain killers as these can mask any of the warnings signs to stop exercising.
4. **Stop** exercising immediately if you feel any pain or twinges.
5. **Stop** exercising if your muscles start to quiver. It is a sign that you are doing too much. Relax, there is always tomorrow.
6. Do not exercise your facial muscles if you feel tired, emotionally upset or if you are hung over because you won't enjoy it and subconsciously you will remember the negative experience. You can change brain plasticity either negatively or positively. Let the brain record the positive repetitive changes only!
7. Be especially cautious with the neck exercises, take it very gently and **totally avoid them** if you experience any discomfort, aches or back problems. Don't bring your head too far back, if it says "tilt your head", that's what it means. It does not mean to thrust your head as far back as humanly possible!
8. When beginning exercising use a mirror initially, unless specifically stated not to do so. When you become proficient at each of the exercises you will no longer need to look in the

mirror, except to ensure that you are continually doing them correctly.

9. Start slowly; get used to each of the exercises. If you find one too difficult at first, leave it out and come back to it later. Your muscle tone will improve over time and therefore, as with any exercise you will be able to do more, eventually. Remember exercising must be fun as well as good for you.

10. Remember that frequency is more important than the length of time spent on **Fitface toning**. Begin with a minimum of 15 minutes every day for the first three months. After that continue with a maintenance programme of 3 to 4 times a week.

11. Remember less is more; do not do more than half an hour of continuous **Fitface toning** exercises in any one day. However, be sensible; when you are learning, understand that what should take 20 minutes may take an hour!

12. Begin gently, if you find either the number of repetitions or the length of the hold time too difficult at first, relax. Move on. Over time, you may gradually work up to the required holding time or number of repetitions. If not, it is not the end of the world, just enjoy your routine.

13. Always relax your shoulders.

14. Always remember to breathe.

15. Maintain a healthy well rounded programme adding in a couple of extra exercises for problem areas in addition to the basic routine. Just as you don't work exclusively on one muscle at the gym, you work the whole body; work your whole face with **Fitface toning.** The exercises are designed to be mixed and matched. **Do not concentrate on just your problem areas or only a few exercises. IT WON'T WORK and this is the biggest mistake most people make.**

16. Eventually learn a **Fitface toning** routine by heart so that you can perform it anywhere, even watching television or in the tub (bath)!

17. Remember this for later. If on the first day, or the second day, or whenever you try **Fitface toning** and your muscles become sore, **stop**. Do not over do it. Come back. Try again. Start over. It is only natural that when you move muscles that have not been used much before, that once stretched they will feel sore. Soon they will rebuild and become stronger, tighter than ever before.

Getting started with Fitface facial toning exercises

What will you need most?
Your ambition!

Change

For most of us starting something new is both scary and exciting. We all react differently to change. Some people fail at the first anxious thought of change, resist and never even get started. Others try with a running start but fall at the first hurdle and just give up! Then there are those who rise to the challenge, grasp hold of their mindset and approach change with vigour embracing the possibilities! The majority of people's attitude to change is to fall somewhere between the two extremes. The only way I can support you through your learning curve is to state that <u>if you don't try, you are guaranteed to fail</u>. Remember this and you are halfway there.

Self discipline

The only way that the toning exercises will work for you is if you do them regularly. You must also enjoy them. If you make them fun and easy, they will be! Plan to do them every day for the first three months and then 3 to 4 times per week. Sticking to a routine is always difficult but rewarding. You will not only look better physically but mentally, you will feel better for the achievement. Pat yourself on the back.

Belief

You must believe that the time, commitment, dedication and effort will pay off. Working out doesn't stop at the neck. **Fitface toning** works. Reread the pages on all the benefits of facial toning or just think about the possible horrors of surgery.

Motivation

Motivation is the <u>**single most important key ingredient**</u> of the successful outcome of any new venture you undertake. Encourage yourself, tell yourself you "love" doing **Fitface toning** exercises and you will. Plan to succeed and you will. Teach your brain to think the right thoughts; you are what you think you are. If you "think" you will, you will, if you think you can't you won't. It's never too late to start. I have included a few inspirational quotes on a separate page for you to turn to when motivation is needed.

Commitment

Facial exercises are not a quick fix. Immediate change in your appearance is not going to be dramatic. Muscular development doesn't happen over night, it is a process, it will take time; please don't give up at the first hurdle. The result of your time, dedication and commitment will have lasting effects.

Dedication

You will need to take **15 or 20 minutes out of everyday** to do these exercises for the first 3 months, you will and can find the time if you really want to. Maybe try to fit in some toning while you watch a TV programme or wait for the washing to dry, whatever, if you want to find the time you will! Later, why not incorporate **Fitface toning** into your work out routine or do facial exercises on alternate days instead of bodywork on your 'off days'.

Concentration

You can learn to move any muscle, it just takes dedication and concentration, tell yourself you can move that muscle and you will, believe, it takes practise. As a child were you not taught to, "Try, try and try again?"

Patience

You will eventually learn the exercises by heart and the routines will only take 15 or 20 minutes, it will not happen over night. It takes time and patience to become proficient. Remember that on the first day you will be exasperated and the routine may end up taking an hour to do just a few exercises. Don't worry, don't be concerned. Ultimately, **Fitface toning** will become second nature to you.

Understanding

Listen to your body, if you think you are doing too much you probably are. If there is any pain or discomfort stop. It's your body talking to you, **listen.** It knows best!

Other things you will need:
1. To consult with your physician if you are in any doubt whatsoever about your personal circumstances as to whether or not you should perform **Fitface toning**.
2. A clean face and neck (no make-up) freshly moisturised.
3. A glass of water.

4. A clock with a second hand.
5. Your hair pulled back away from the face.
6. A mirror, initially on a table.
7. A chair.

You are now ready to begin on improving and toning the already beautiful you. Whatever you need to do to succeed, **just do it** (as now coined by **Nike**). If you need to write these inspirational, thought provoking motivational sayings down, buy the posters, memorise these phrases and stick them in your bathroom, do whatever it takes.

Inspirational quotes

My personal favourite is my school motto

Beyond the best, there is a better!

Winners

While most are dreaming of success, winners, wake-up
and work hard to achieve it.

Only number 1 is remembered, don't settle for second place.

Success

You have to think you can win.
You have to feel you can win.
You have to believe you can win.
You have to know you can win.
You have to be certain - that winning is the only option.

Goals

Have one only.
Be single minded in your approach.

Challenge

Relish the thought of new experiences to stretch yourself
to your full potential.
Get out of your comfort zone!

Commitment

When the going gets tough, the tough get going.

Sorts the winners, from the losers.

Perseverance

The difference between a successful person and others:
it is not, a lack of strength,
it is not, a lack of knowledge
but is, rather a lack of will.

Determination

I will do it.
Failure is not an option.

Fitface toning training programmes

Basic

The **Fitface toning** training programme begins with a basic introductory easy **Fitface toning** programme. This programme is what it says it is a **Basic,** no nonsense anytime, everywhere routine that is suitable for anyone. The basic programme can done by anyone without any training or learning. The other programmes require more effort and need to be learnt and practised.

There are three different **Fitface toning** training programmes, beginning with the **Anytime Fitface** toning programme at the beginner's level, advancing through to the **Standard Fitface** toning programme and finishing with the **Advanced Fitface** toning routine. A 3 step programme, built for you to gently work through at your own pace. Each programme is designed for a different stage of your personal development, with 3 separate and distinct levels within each programme to progress through.

Additionally, there is a **Micro Fitface toning** workout for when time is very short which only takes 3 minutes.

Programmes

Step 1 Anytime   **Fitface Programme**
Step 2 Standard   **Fitface Programme**
Step 3 Advanced   **Fitface Programme**

+ Micro Fitface toning
Within the 3 step programme, there are 3 separate levels of attainment possible within each routine.

Levels

1. **Beginner's level**
2. **Regular level**
3. **Target level**

   +Extra Exercises only available at the Advanced Level

   - **Beginner's level** is the basic, entry level at which to start performing each of the new programmes.
   - **Regular level** is the next or the second level of expertise, for each programme.
   - **Target level** is the final upper, third level of attainment to targeted for your own unique specific facial areas that you wish to improve.
   - **Extra Exercises** are at the Advanced Level and only for the determined and dedicated.

Target

Each exercise has a target zone; this is the area of the face that the exercise is primarily working on. However, do remember that the muscles of the face all work in conjunction with one another, so you exercise one, you exercise them all. The target is only a guide to help you to target your problem areas. I stress, do not target just a few exercises, Fitface is not designed to work like that. If you strengthen one muscle exclusively another will suffer and that is, in my opinion how the fascia literately gets stuck in a groove as explained fully in **Chapter 2**.

Be patient with yourself

The brain is a remarkable organ, it has the ability to make new connections every second, constantly evolving and altering due to its plasticity and memory. Because of this, you have the power to change at any time. The more repetition an action, the more proficient you will become at it, just like riding a bike or learning a dance routine, so it is with **Fitface toning**.

At first it may be difficult, your muscles may need to strengthen in order to do some of the exercises and in time they will, but don't give up, try, try and try again. As those new connections in the brain are made, the evolution occurs and in time, the various exercises will become second nature to you as your muscles learn what you require of them. The most important thing to remember is that learning any new routine takes time until you become totally familiar with it. Please don't get frustrated with any of the **Fitface facial toning exercises**, if you can't master a pose, move on and come back to it another day. You must enjoy what you're doing.

In the beginning it will take you much, much longer to do any of the programmes. You will be looking at the book, looking at yourself, trying to master your performance and it will seem to take ages, but eventually you won't even need a mirror, and then only the **Fitface toning** guide to refresh your memory. Just remember, although you might not be able to do an exercise today, tomorrow you will. It just takes time. Practise makes perfect.

Photos

I encourage everyone to take "before and after" **Fitface** photographs. However, don't expect miracles, those only happen when the photos are touched up professionally or the lighting has been changed deliberately for celebrities or advertisements. Be realistic. Take one at the start, another about 4 months later, another at 7 months and finally a photo at a year. The photos should be taken in the same place, at about the same time, with the same lighting conditions. I would love to see the results. Do bear in mind that a year later, without **Fitface toning** you would normally have looked older, you will be amazed at the results.

Beginning

Although facial muscles work as a team, each of the twenty-six voluntary muscles of the face should be trained separately. The facial exercise instructions start with a warm up and then flow down the face, from the forehead to the neck. This order is important, not critical but I suggest you follow it.

Maintenance

For maximum results, I would recommend that you **exercise 5 times weekly or daily,** (with weekends off) **for the first three months** and **then, follow a maintenance** routine of **every other day,** alternating between <u>all</u> the different routines. However, be sensible, if your muscles are tired skip a day or two. Only do what you can. Remember that pain is a sign to stop as well as quivering muscles.

Experience has shown me and my clients that it is better to learn one programme thoroughly (in order that your muscles learn what is required of them) before even attempting to progress to the next programme or level. But even when you have completed the last programme at the advanced level, I would still suggest that you keep mixing up your programmes (depending on your mood) to give yourself a totally balanced look.

Mix and Match (IMPORTANT)

Personally, I tend to do, what I feel, when I feel like it For example; I do the **Advanced Fitface toning programme** when I'm feeling brilliant and energetic, the **Anytime Fitface toning programme** when I'm on holiday, travelling etc (because it's the easiest to remember) and the **Standard Fitface toning programme** most of the time. I also throw in some of the **Basic Fitface exercises** whenever I can. It's all a matter of choice. It is your choice, the most important thing is just to enjoy. DON'T FEEL GUILTY IF YOU MISS A DAY, a week, or even a month. Begin again. Try, try and try again, don't ever just give up for good! On the other hand don't keep procrastinating that you will start tomorrow. **Start today.**

The Fitface 3 steps programme

Commence with the **Basic Fitface**. It's fundamental, the foundations, it is also fun, it's easy and it's a start. When you are familiar with the exercises (a minimum of a week, or having completed all the exercises easily at least five times) and you want to move on to the real programme, begin with the real programme. If not, no worries, you can stay with Basic **Fitface** forever, diving in and out whenever you like, some facial exercise is better than no facial exercise.

Step 1
- **Anytime Fitface toning programme**

This routine was designed to be done anywhere, (watching TV, listening to the radio, in the tub (bath), in the dark as a passenger in a car/train/coach/plane journey) at anytime.

Eventually, you will be able to perform the programme without the use of a mirror. It's simple and super effective. This programme should be **practised for a minimum of a month** before continuing to the next programme, ideally at least six weeks.

Step 2
- **Standard Fitface toning programme**

This routine was designed to be the next stage up from the **Anytime Fitface toning programme** and therefore should not be attempted until the Regular level of the **Anytime Fitface toning programme** has been achieved and maintained for six weeks.

The previous routine has allowed your muscles to learn, build and become more familiar with some of the **Fitface toning** exercises before introducing more complicated movements. **Maintain for 6 weeks** after which you may want to progress to the next programme, but do what you can. Stay at this level for life if you prefer.

Step 3
- **Advanced Fitface toning programme**

This routine was designed to be the next step up from the **Standard Fitface toning programme** and therefore should not be attempted until the Regular level has been achieved and **maintained for more than six weeks.** The previous programme has enabled your muscles to become familiar with complex movements and promoted new muscles growth. Eventually you will be able to master the Advanced programme at the Standard level and if you wish also Target specific areas.

The **Fitface toning** programmes routines should all be used in conjunction with one another to give your facial muscles balance. The idea of the 3 step **Fitface** facial exercise routine is to give your face tone and build muscle mass.

That's it!

Exercise professionals or fanatics (only for the toughest - not me)!
If you are a professional one of those super fit young ladies (that I see at the gym 24/7) and would like to take **Fitface toning** to the max, in the shortest amount of time, then I would suggest that you learn each programme for only a month. Then continue with a 5 times a week maintenance routine at the Target level, a routine in which every other workout is the **Advanced Fitface toning programme.**

Problem areas
You may want to put extra toning emphasis on an area or areas that concerns you. You can easily accomplish this by choosing up to 3 extra exercises that target your problem area and incorporate them into any of the programmes, **see the Target level of each routine.** However, remember to work out at the less intense levels initially and to refrain from spot building (targeting an area exclusively). Do not add more than 5 minutes a day by targeting an area.

Advanced optional extras
These **Extra Exercises** were designed for those persons who have reached the **Target Level of the Advanced Programme** and STILL want additional choices with their problem areas.

Micro Fitface toning programme

When you have no time at all, or you are on holiday, give yourself a 3 minute micro work out every other day at the bare minimum. Everyday would be even better.

This is the most important exercise in the whole of the **Fitface toning programmes** and therefore it is present within each one. It is an isometric exercise, that is very difficult to learn but once mastered, this toning exercise can be performed at anytime, anywhere.

The first exercise in the **BASIC FITFACE is the "Face-lift".**

1. With eyes open (easier) or shut
2. Lift eyebrows
3. Contract muscle of scalp and temples, lifting your eyebrows up and back to connect with the back of the neck

   - Hold for 1 minute
   - Repeat twice (i.e. for a total of 3 times/minutes)
   -

Note: Feel the whole face pull taut, up and back. Imagine that your whole skull is being tightened, lifted and pulled back.

Tip: Ensure that the sides of your mouth are level with the corners slightly turning up. **DO NOT FROWN**

TARGET Whole face, especially forehead and cheekbones

Daily life tips for a firmer face
- Relax when you are thinking, don't permanently frown
- Hold an exaggerated smile for a minute or two every day. Not only will this make you look better but you will feel better too!
- Once you have totally learned a **Fitface** routine you have the ideal opportunity to "multi task", try doing some isometric exercises at the same time. While doing some of the easier **Fitface toning** exercises try to tighten your abs, legs or buttocks and pull your shoulders back all at the same time!
- Once you become proficient at the toning exercise it's also a great time to tone those internal muscles

- Remember, everyone progresses at a different rate. An exercise that is difficult for one person might be easy for another, accept this, it is just the way we are all made slightly differently and **Fitface** is not a competition. It should only be performed to make you feel better about yourself.

Programmes duration

This depends totally on how familiar you are with the exercises. In broad terms I think of each exercise as taking approximately 1 minute. Each programme has 14/15 exercises with the **Micro** or **Face-lift** taking only 3 minutes. Therefore I would expect you to spend approximately 20 minutes on each programme.

Chapter 7

BASIC FITFACE
1 Face-lift

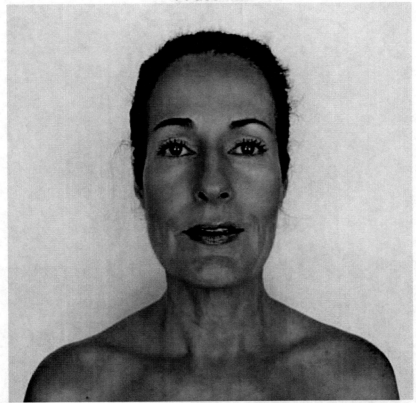

TARGET Whole face, especially forehead and cheekbones

1. With eyes open (easier) or better shut
2. Lift eyebrows
3. Contract muscle of scalp and temples, lifting you eyebrows up and back to connect with the back of the neck
- Hold for I minute
- Repeat twice (i.e. for a for a total of 3 times)

Note:
Feel the whole face pull taut, up and back. Imagine that your whole skull is being tightened, lifted and pulled back.
Tip:
Ensure that the sides of your mouth are level with the corners slightly turning up. **DO NOT FROWN**

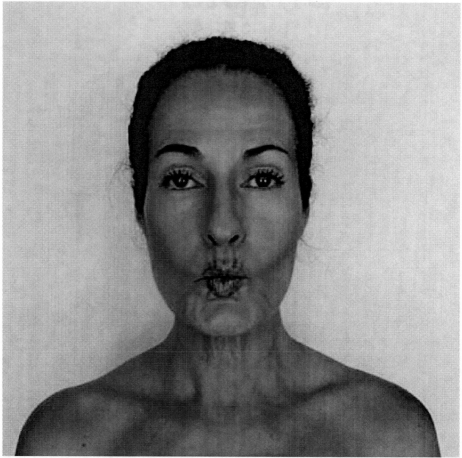

TARGET Forehead, lips, *nasolabial* folds

1. With closed lips, move lips forward into a kiss
2. Lift eyebrows high

- Hold for 1 minute

BASIC
3 Puffers

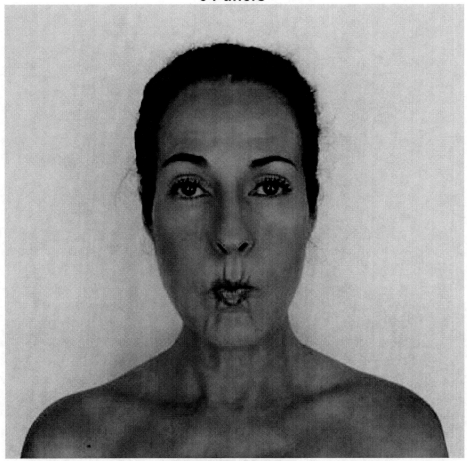

TARGET Cheeks

1. Blow up cheeks with air
2. Lift eyebrows (if you want an extra pull)

- Hold for 1 minute

BASIC
4 Grimaces

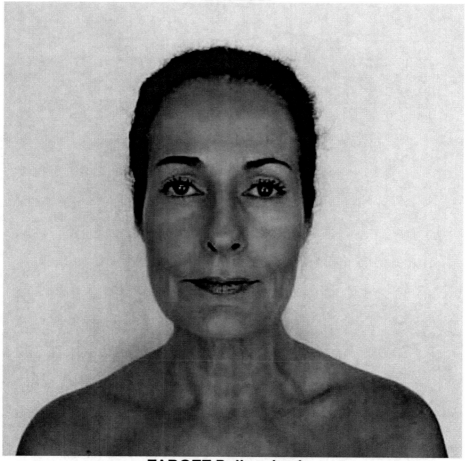

TARGET Pull up jowls

1. Lips closed, make a broad straight smile
2. Lift eyebrows (if you want an extra pull)

- Hold for 1 minute

BASIC
5 Happy smiles

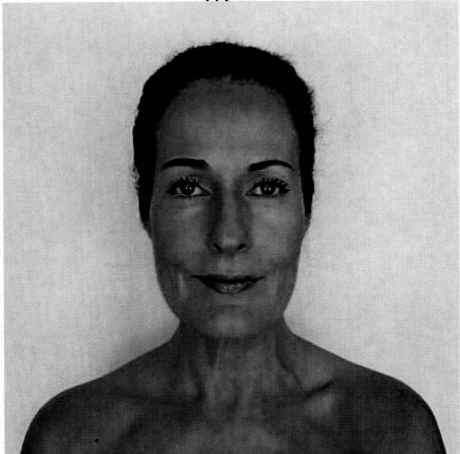

TARGET Pull up jowls, lift lower face

1. Lips closed, make a broad smile and extend to the earlobes
2. Lift eyebrows (if you want an extra pull)

- Hold for 1 minute

BASIC
6 Laughs

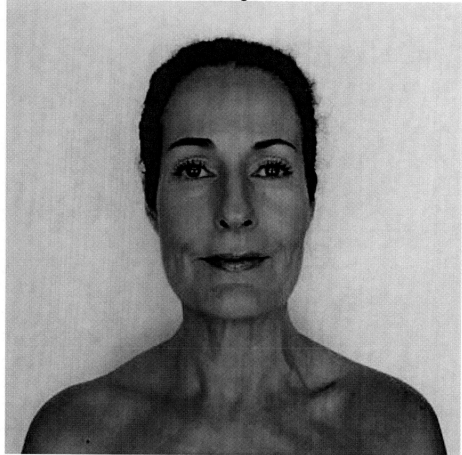

TARGET Jowls and face-lift and under eye

1. Lips closed, make a big broad smile, huge smile right up to the corners of the eyes – yes, showing crow's feet!
2. Lift eyebrows (if you want an extra pull)

- Hold for 1 minute

Note:
Your lips will want to part but don't let them.

BASIC
7 Snarls

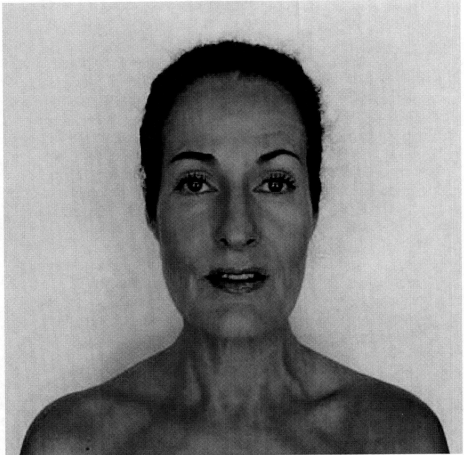

TARGET Cheeks and nasolabial folds

1. Begin with lips closed and raise your top lip only avoid the bottom lips natural tendency to pull downward, instead try to keep the bottom lip straight)
2. Lift eyebrows (if you want an extra pull)

• Hold for 1 minute

Note:
Try to feel the outer top of the snarl being pulled up by the temple.

BASIC
8 Flutters

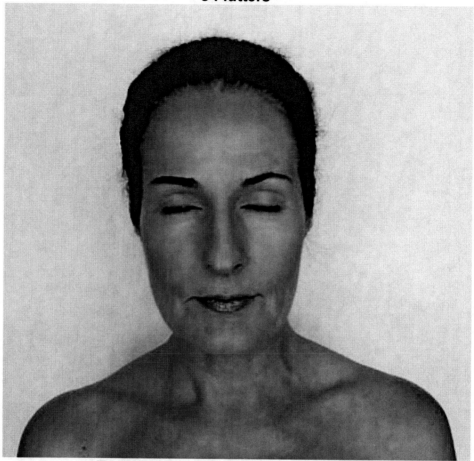

TARGET Inner and outer eye corners

1. Flutter your eyelashes as quickly as possible, completely opening and closing the eye i.e. very rapid blinks
2. Lift eyebrows (if you want an extra pull)

- Continue for 1 minute

BASIC
9 Winks

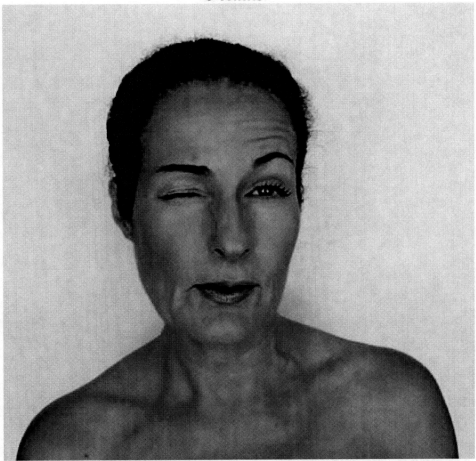

TARGET Crows feet and frown lines

1. Keep one eye open and the other shut and wink fully on one side
2. Repeat with the other eye

• 30 repetitions each eye. Approximately 1 minute total exercise

Note:
If you should find that one eye is stronger than the other, or you can wink with one eye but not the other, practise more with the weaker eye. For example do 45 repetitions on the weak eye and only 15 on the stronger eye.

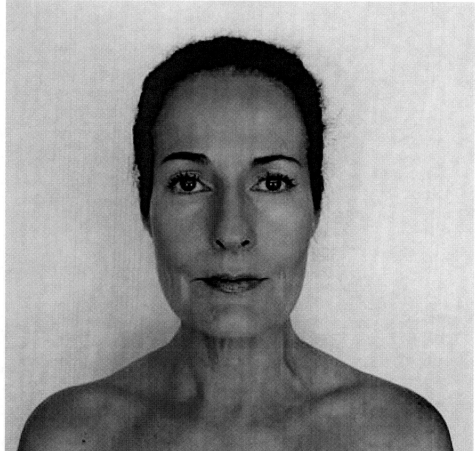

TARGET Frown lines, eye tendons and muscles around the eyes

1. Open your eyes wide and stare at a distance object
2. Hold as long as you can. Blink, when you have to and start again

- Continue doing this for approximately 1 minute

BASIC
11 Moons

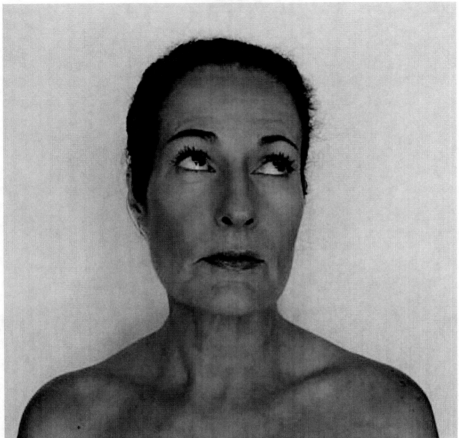

TARGET Temples, frown lines and tendons of the eye

1. Look as far as possible to one side, and circle eyes upwards looking at the tops of your eyebrows and round over and down to the opposite side
2. Lift the eyes and circle upwards to the opposite side.

• Continue doing this for approximately 1 minute

Note:
It feels like making crescent moons repeatedly from side to side.

BASIC
12 Pouches

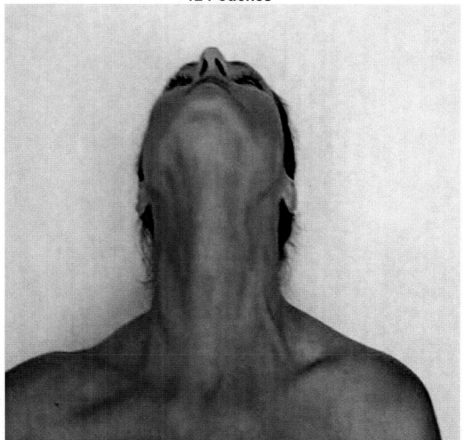

TARGET Neck, jowls & under chin

1. Ensure that your neck is long and relaxed before gently dropping your head backwards
2. Push your tongue up into the roof of your mouth.
3. Hold for approximately 20 seconds, release your tongue
4. Bring your head into the upright position

• Repeat twice

Note:
You may not be able to hold this position for 20 seconds. For example: If you can only manage a 10 second hold, just repeat the exercise four times instead of a total of 3 times.

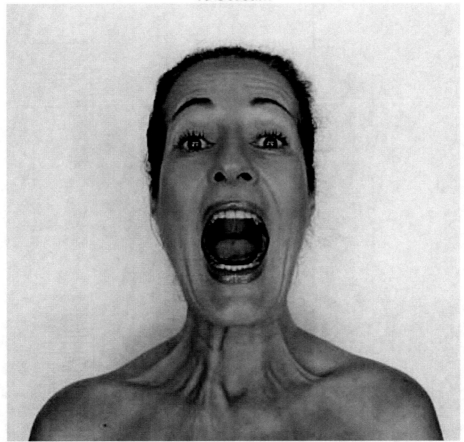

TARGET Everything, whole face.

1. Make a scream (without making a noise)

•   Hold taut for 1 minute

Note:
If this is too much, hold for 30 seconds and repeat. You should feel the whole face come alive and feel as if it has been fully stretched.

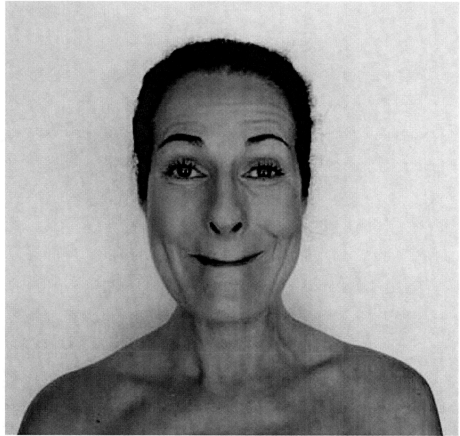

TARGET Cheeks, under eye area & eyebrows

1. Pull top lip over teeth
2. Push bottom jaw forward and pull bottom lip over teeth
3. Pull up sides of nose, cheeks

- Hold continuously for approximately 1 minute

Note:
This is difficult and may take you a while to master, start with holding for less time and work up to 1 minute.

Chapter 8

Step 1

Anytime Fitface toning programme

The **Anytime Fitface toning** programme was designed to be your introduction to **Fitface toning**, to be done anywhere (whilst watching TV, listening to the radio, in the bath) at anytime. The Anytime **Fitface toning** programme is relatively easy to learn. Once learnt you will be able to complete the programme without a mirror! It's a simple and super effective programme at the Regular level.

Do not progress to the next stage (Standard) until you have allowed your muscles to build and become familiar with some of the basic toning exercises before introducing those more complex movements. The routine should be used in conjunction with the other programmes to give your face a balanced training routine. The idea of the 3 step **Fitface toning** programme is to give your face a toned appearance.

There are three levels to progress through: Beginners, Regular and Target. The first two levels in each programme must be completed before continuing to the next programme stage. The Target level of each programme is optional; it is the Regular level but more intense with the opportunity to select additional exercises to target your own personal problem areas.

Beginner's level

Week one
Either cut the repetitions or the duration of each exercise in half.
Only when you are ready, continue to the next **Regular level.**

Regular level

Continue with the full programme for the next six weeks.
Only when you are ready, continue to the last target level of the programme or change to the Standard **Fitface toning** programme.

Target level

Select any 3 additional toning exercises from:
The Anytime, Standard or Advanced Fitface toning programmes, which you
feel would be the most beneficial for you, to target your personal problem areas.

Notes:

Timings: are for guidance only
Count: means timing in approximate seconds

Duration

This depends totally on how familiar you are with the exercises. In round terms I think of each exercise as taking approximately 1 minute. Each programme has 14/15 exercises with the **Micro** or **Face-lift** taking 3 minutes. Therefore I would expect you to spend approximately 20 minutes on each programme for maximum results.

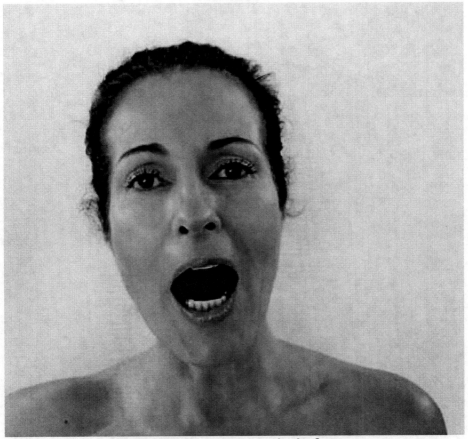

TARGET Warm up - whole face

1. Open your mouth fairly wide
2. Commence an exaggerated circular motion i.e. with your jaw forwards, then downwards, backwards, then upwards rolling forwards

- Repeat continuously for 30 rotations in one direction and then reverse, and continue with 30 movements in the other direction
- Total 1 minute

Note:
Feel as if, you are creating chewing circles forward; then reverse, backwards

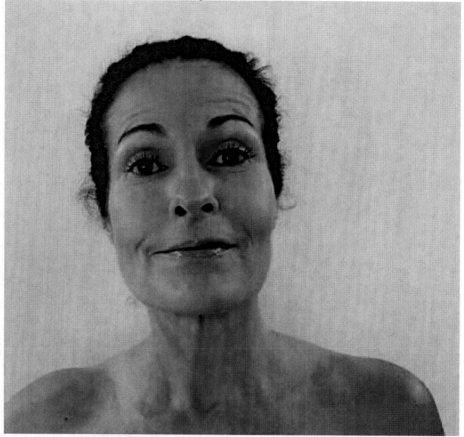

TARGET Brow, eyebrows & upper eyelid

1. Smile gently and hold
2. Lift your eyebrows as high as possible and pause for a couple of seconds
3. Relax

- Repeat approximately 30 times
- Total 1 minute

Note:
Feel as if, you are raising and lowering your eyebrows slowly.

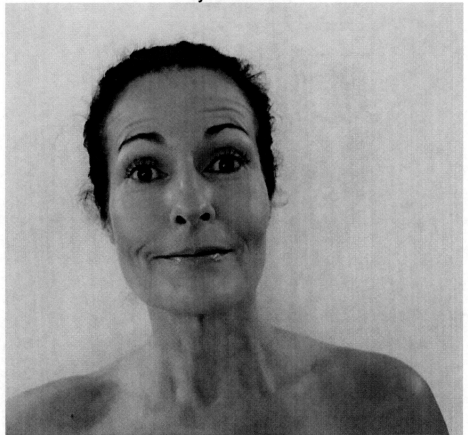

TARGET Brow, eyebrows & upper eyelid

1. Smile gently and hold
2. Lift your eyebrows as high as possible

• Hold for 1 minute

Note:
If this is too long for you, reduce the time by half and repeat twice.

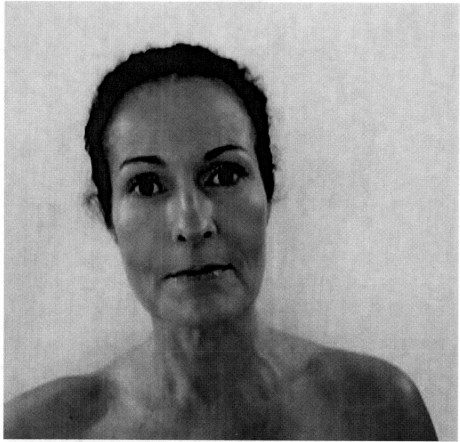

TARGET Whole face, especially forehead and cheekbones

1. With eyes open (easier) or better shut
2. Lift eyebrows
3. Contract muscle of scalp and temples, lifting you eyebrows up and back to connect with the back of the neck.
- Hold for I minute
- Repeat twice (i.e. for a for a total of 3 times)

Note:
Feel the whole face pull taut, up and back. Imagine that your whole skull is being tightened, lifted and pulled back.

Tip:
Ensure that the sides of your mouth are level with the corners slightly turning up. **DO NOT FROWN**

ANYTIME
5 Eye pulls

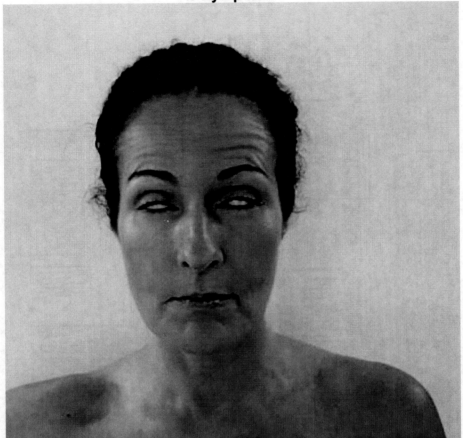

TARGET All around the eyes, both corners, plus under eyelids

1. Begin with eyes shut firmly
2. Raise the eyebrows
3. Try to open your eyes very slowly, for a count of approximately 20 seconds
4. When almost fully open, hold for a count of 10
5. Relax

- Repeat

Note:
This is a difficult exercise to master but you will feel those bags lifting.

ANYTIME
6 Eye clocks

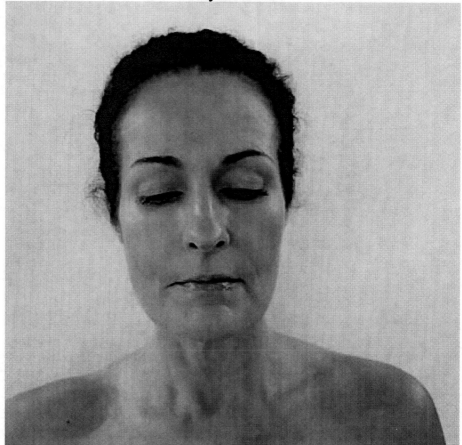

TARGET All around the eyes, both corners, plus under eyelids

1. Lift your eyes up and rotate slowly clockwise for 3 revolutions
2. Repeat anticlockwise

Note:
Each revolution should take about 10 seconds. Extend your glance fully in each direction.

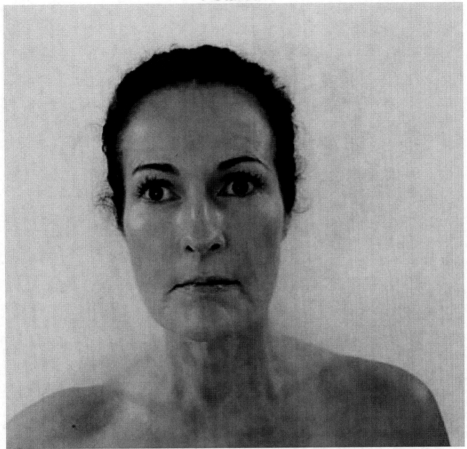

TARGET Eyes, temples & cheeks

1. Open your eyes wide and stare at a distance object
2. Hold as long as you can blink, when you have, relax
3. Start again.
4.
- Continue doing this for approximately 1 minute

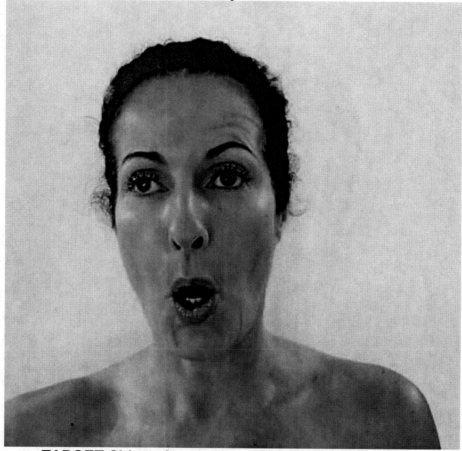

ANYTIME
8 Bunny noses

TARGET Sides of nose, nasolabial folds & upper lip

1. Open your mouth slightly and crinkle your nose
2. Slowly make forward circular motions, up forwards, down and around with the tip of your nose and top lip

- Repeat 20 times in one direction and then reverse
- Continue doing this for approximately 1 minute

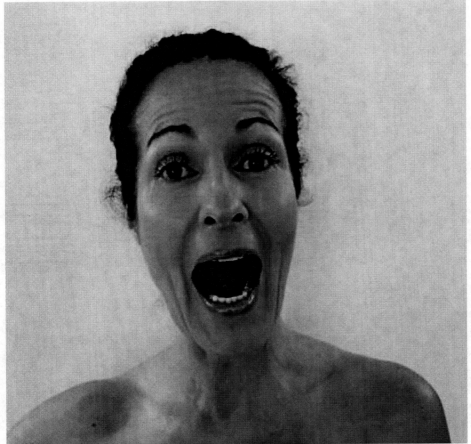

TARGET Lips, cheeks & neck

1. Open your mouth wide and slowly say the vowels A, E, I, O, U in an exaggerated manner

- Repeat 10 times

Note:
You should feel a stretch with each new movement.

ANYTIME
10 Widest smile (showing teeth)

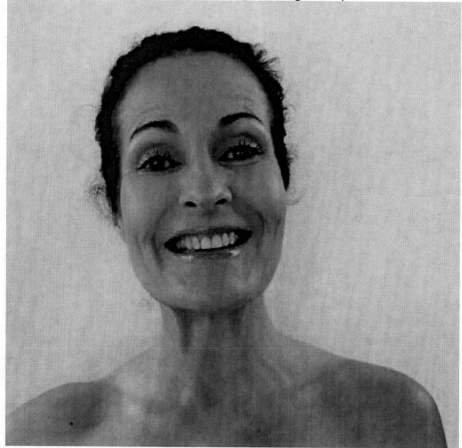

TARGET Cheeks, jowls & chin

1. Make a huge happy broad smile, parting your lips, pulling the lips as wide open to the sides as they will go
2. Lift eyebrows

- Hold wide open for 1 minute

Note:
The smile should extend to the corners of your eyes.

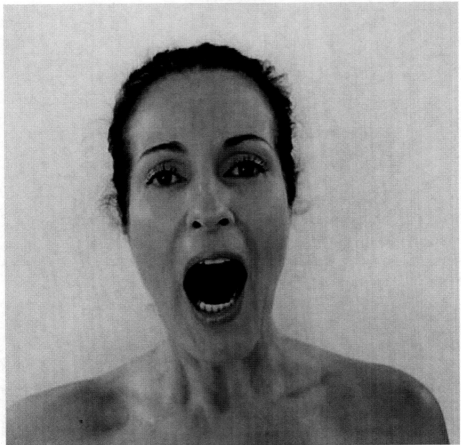

TARGET Cheeks & jowls

1. Open your mouth
2. Smile slightly
3. Chew in reverse slowly with a wide open mouth

- Repeat 50 times

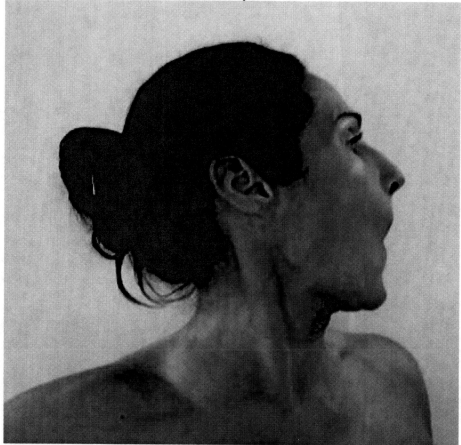

TARGET Jowls & nasolabial folds

1. Turn your head to one side
2. Pull your lips to that side
3. Open and close your mouth slowly but continuously 10 times
4. Relax

- Repeat to the other side

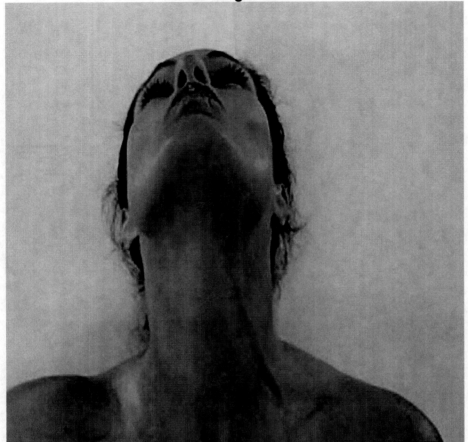

TARGET Neck, chin & sides of mouth

1. Sit upright, feet square, relax your shoulders
2. With your mouth closed, gently extend your neck before tilting your head backwards and let it rest
3. Look at the ceiling
4. Pucker your lips and slowly extend them upwards as if to kiss the ceiling
5. Hold for a count of 10
6. Relax
7. Bring your head slowly forward

- Repeat 3 times

Note:

You will feel this in your neck and possibly your cheeks.

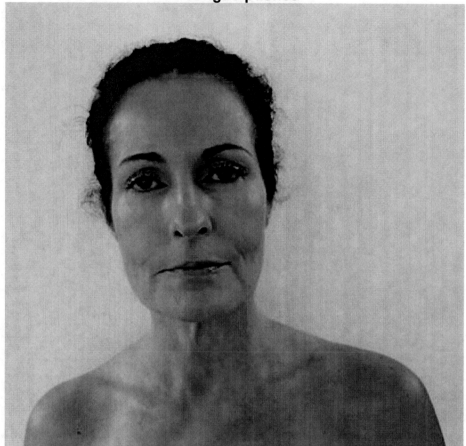

TARGET Under chin

1. With closed lips and teeth gently clench
2. Push your tongue up into the roof of your mouth.
3. Hold for approximately 30 seconds, release your tongue, relax

• Repeat once

Note:
You should feel the muscles under your chin and at the sides of the jaw working.

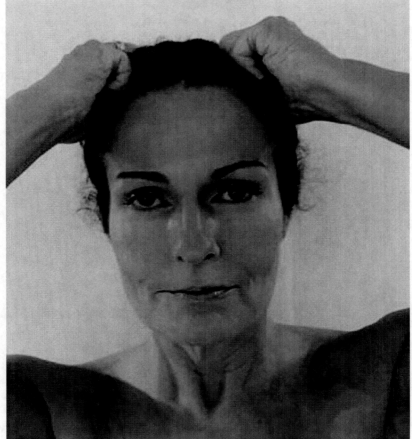

TARGET Scalp & everywhere!

1. Grasp your hair by the roots at the temples
2. Gently, firmly pull the hair making small slow circular rotations
3. Make 3 clockwise rotations and then another three circles anti-clockwise
4. Move your hands a little further away and repeat

- Continue moving your hands over your scalp for about a minute

Chapter 9

Step 2

Standard Fitface toning programme

The **Standard** routine was designed to be the next stage up from the Anytime **Fitface toning** programme and to be the intermediate programme. Therefore this stage should not be attempted until the Anytime programme has been achieved and maintained for more than six weeks. This will allow your muscles to build and become familiar with some of the fundamental toning exercises before introducing these more complex movements.

Do not progress to the next programme (Advanced) until you have given your muscles a chance to become accustomed to the new programme which generally takes a month. The routine should be used in conjunction with the other programmes to give your face a balanced training routine. The idea of the 3 step **Fitface toning** programme is to give your face toned appearance, not a body builder's taut face.

There are three levels to progress through: Beginners, Regular and Target. The first two levels in each programme must be completed before continuing to the next stage. The Target level of each programme is optional; it is the Regular level but more intense with the opportunity to select additional exercises to target your own personal problem areas.

Beginner's level

Week one
Either cut the repetitions or the duration of each exercise in half.
<u>Only when you are ready,</u> continue to the next **Regular level.**

Regular level

Continue with the full programme for the next six weeks.
<u>Only when you are ready</u>, continue to the last target level of the programme or change to the Standard **Fitface toning** programme.

Target level

Select any 3 additional toning exercises from:
The Anytime, Standard or Advanced **Fitface toning** programmes, which you feel would be most beneficial for you, to target your personal problem areas.

Notes:

Timings: are for guidance only
Count: means timing in approximate seconds

Duration

This depends totally on how familiar you are with the exercises. In round terms I think of each exercise as taking approximately 1 minute. Each programme has 14/15 exercises with the **Micro** or **Face-lift** taking 3 minutes. Therefore I would expect you to spend approximately 20 minutes on each programme for maximum results.

STANDARD
1 Big O kiss

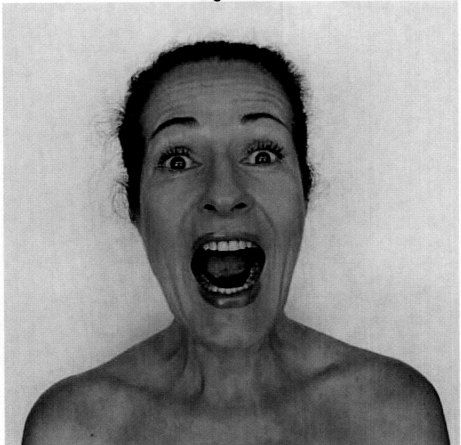

TARGET Warm up - whole face

1. Open your mouth as wide as you can
2. Raise your eyebrows (pulling everything back)
3. Pause for a moment
4. Slowly bring your lips in to form a kiss with your eyebrows into a slight frown
5. Pause for a moment

- Repeat continuously for 20 repetitions

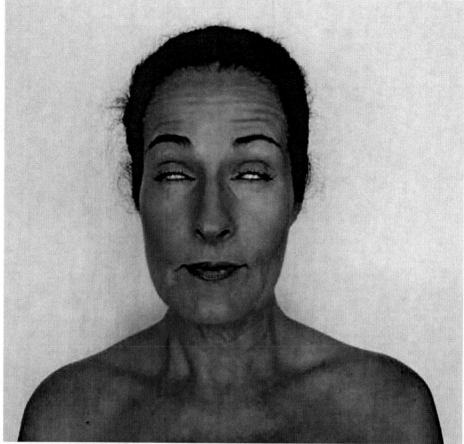

TARGET Brow, eyebrows & upper eyelid

1. Close your eyes
2. Raise your eyebrows as high as possible and then lower slowly but continuously

- Repeat 30 times
- Total 1 minute

Note:
Resist the urge to open your eyes. Should they open momentarily as mine have, just close them again.

STANDARD
3 Face-lift

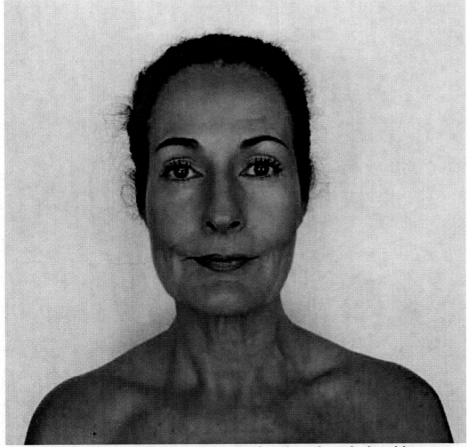

TARGET Whole face, especially forehead and cheekbones

1. With eyes open (easier) or shut
2. Lift eyebrows
3. Contract muscle of scalp and temples, lifting you eyebrows up and back to connect with the back of the neck

- Hold for I minute
- Repeat twice (i.e. for a total of 3 times)

Note:
Feel the whole face pull taut, up and back. Imagine that your whole skull is being tightened, lifted and pulled back.
Tip: Ensure that the sides of your mouth are level with the corners slightly turning up. **DO NOT FROWN**

179

STANDARD
4 Stares

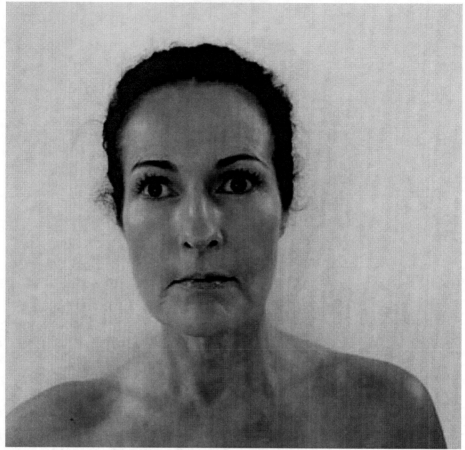

TARGET Eyes, temples & cheeks

1. Open your eyes wide and stare at a distance object.
2. Hold as long as you can. Blink, when you have to and start again

- Continue doing this for approximately 1 minute

STANDARD
5 Eye pulls

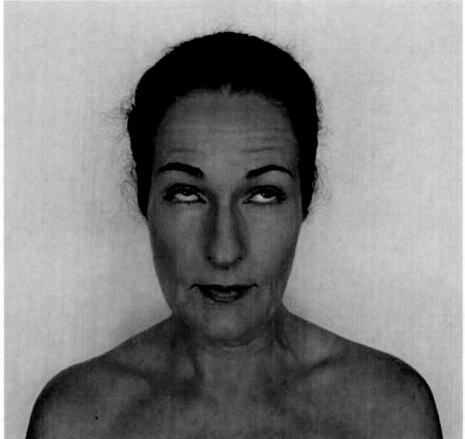

TARGET All around the eyes: both corners, plus under eyelids

1. Begin with eyes shut firmly
2. Raise the eyebrows
3. Try to open your eyes very slowly, for a count of approximately 20 seconds
4. When almost fully open, hold for a count of 10
5. Relax

• Repeat

Note:
This is a difficult exercise to master but you will feel those bags lifting.

STANDARD
6 Eye clocks

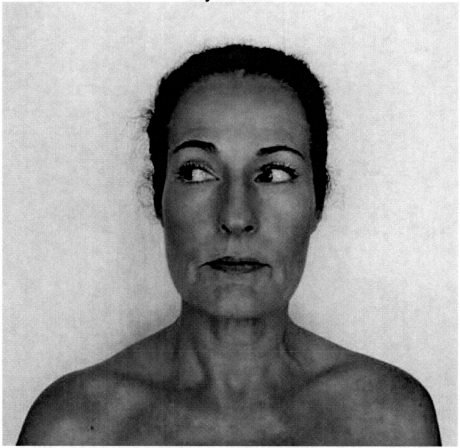

TARGET All around the eyes:
inner & outer corners, plus under eyelids

1. Lift your eyes up and rotate slowly clockwise for 3 revolutions
2. Repeat anticlockwise

Note:
Each revolution should take about 10 seconds. Extend your glance fully in each direction.

STANDARD
7 Bunny noses

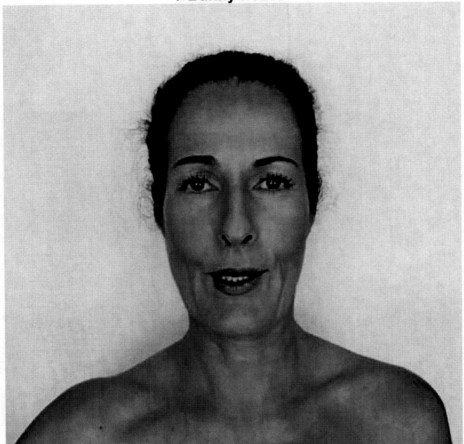

TARGET Sides of nose, nasolabial folds & upper lip

1. Open your mouth slightly and crinkle your nose
2. Slowly make forward circular motions, up forwards, down and around with the tip of your nose and top lip

- Repeat 20 times in one direction and then reverse
  Continue doing this for approximately1minute

STANDARD
8 Three smiles

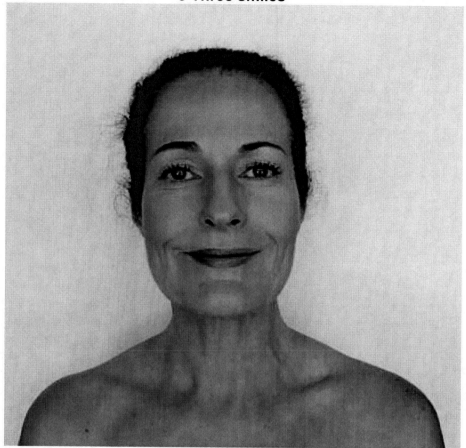

TARGET Cheeks & jowls

1. Lips together smile horizontally, hold count to 10
2. Lips together smile more towards the earlobes, hold count to 10
3. Lips together make a huge smile towards the temples, hold count to 10
4. Still holding taut, reverse each move - i.e. smile towards the earlobes and hold for a count of 10

- Repeat
  i.e. smile horizontally and hold for a count of 10
  i.e. smile towards the earlobes and hold for a count of 10

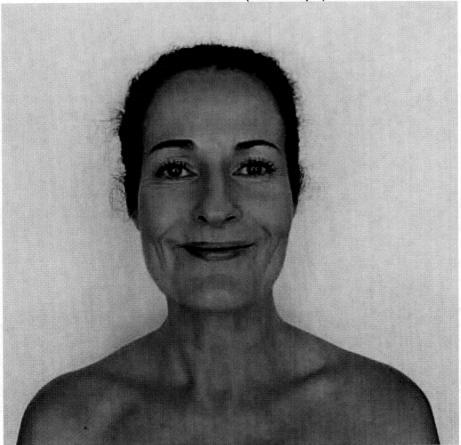

TARGET Cheeks, jowls & chin

1. Make a huge happy broad smile, with closed lips, pulling the lips as wide open to the sides as they will go.
2. Lift eyebrows

• Hold wide open for I minute

Note:
The smile should extend to the corners of your eyes.

STANDARD
10 Nose pulls

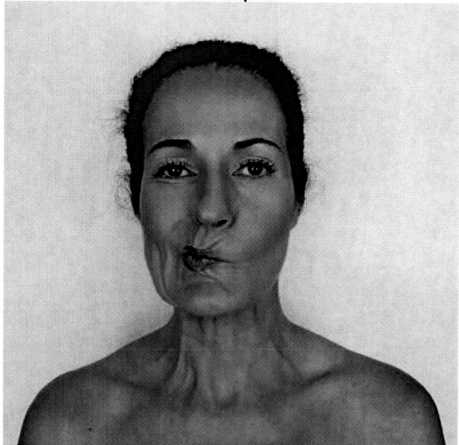

TARGET Lips and cheeks

1. Pucker your lips into a pursed kiss
2. Very slowly pull them as far to one side of the face as you can comfortably, pause, but do not release the tension
3. Still holding your lips taut move them to the other side of the face, the corner of the mouth should be turned upwards

• Repeat 6 times

Note:
This is difficult, you may have to stop half way and release the tension and start again.

STANDARD
11 Tongue out

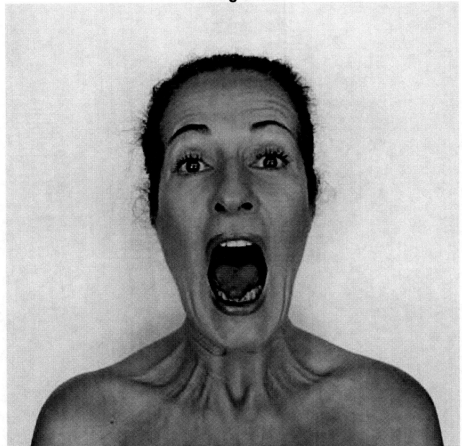

TARGET Lips, neck & chin

1. Open your mouth as wide as possible
2. Stick your tongue out as far as possible
3. Raise you eyebrows
- Hold for a count of 25

- Repeat

Note:
There may be a tendency to pull the lips forward after a while, try to resist by pulling them up as if smiling at the corners of the mouth. This is harder than it looks, be patient with yourself, only hold for a count of 15 at first, don't over strain.

STANDARD
12 Jowl pull smile

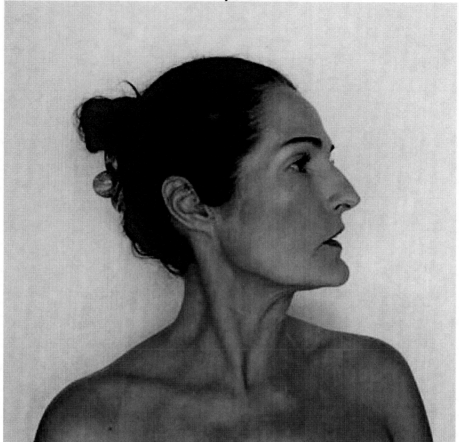

TARGET Jowls & nasolabial folds

1. Turn your head to one side
2. Open your mouth slightly
3. Pull your lips to that side; they should automatically pull up to the temple, pause and hold taut for a count of 30
4. Relax

- Repeat to the other side

STANDARD
13 Jaw circles

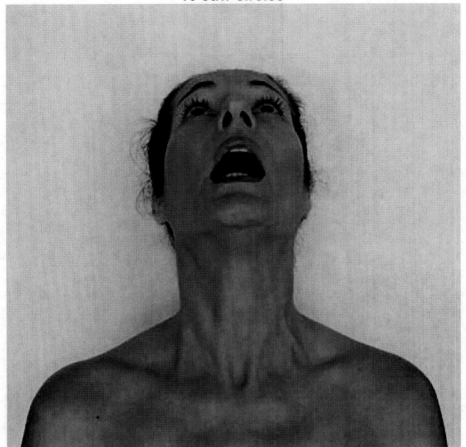

TARGET Chin & neck

1. Sit upright, relax your shoulders with feet firmly planted on the floor
2. Extend your neck and gently tilt your head backwards looking at the ceiling in front of you
3. Open your mouth wide and start a slow chewing movement forwards 10 times
4. Pause and reverse movement, chewing backwards slowly 10 times
5. Slowly bring your head to an upright position

- Repeat

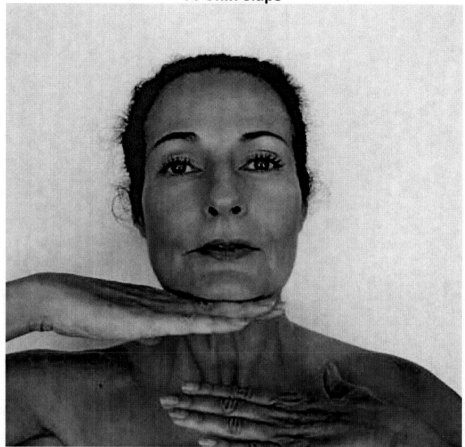

TARGET Jowls & cheeks

1. With the backs of your hands, firmly slap the underneath of your chin, following your jaw line from one side to the other side and back again

*   Repeat continuously for about a minute

STANDARD
15 Ears relaxation

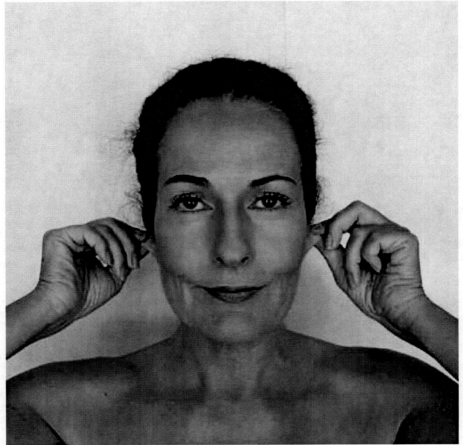

TARGET Ears & jowls

1. Pinch your earlobes and massage between fingers moving up the back of the ear coming all the way to the front
2. Put your index finger in your ear hole and gently rotate your finger to massage inner ear whilst your thumb gently massages the back of the outer ear

Chapter 10

Step 3

Advanced Fitface toning programme

The Advanced routine was designed to be the next stage up from the Standard **Fitface toning** programme and the last stage. Therefore this stage should not be attempted until the Standard programme has been achieved and maintained for at least six weeks. This will allow your muscles to build and become familiar with some of the central toning exercises before introducing these more complicated movements.

This routine should be used in conjunction with all the other programmes to give your face a balanced training routine. The idea of the 3 step **Fitface** is to give your face a toned appearance.

There are three levels to progress through: Beginners, Regular and Target. The first two levels in each programme must be completed before continuing to the next stage. The Target level of each programme is optional; it is the Regular level but more intense with the opportunity to select additional exercises to target your own personal problem areas.

Beginner's level

Week one
Either cut the repetitions or the duration in half for each exercise.
<u>Only when you are ready,</u> continue to the next **Regular level**.

Regular level

Continue with the full programme for the next six weeks.
<u>Only when you are ready</u>, continue to the last target level.

Target level

Select any 3 additional toning exercises from:
The Anytime, Standard or Advanced **Fitface toning** programmes

which you feel would be the most beneficial for you, to target your personal problem areas.

Notes:

Timings: are for guidance only
Count: means approximate seconds

Duration

This depends totally on how familiar you are with the exercises. In round terms I think of each exercise as taking approximately 1 minute. Each programme has 14/15 exercises with the **Micro** or **Face-lift** taking 3 minutes. Therefore I would expect you to spend approximately 20 minutes on each programme for maximum results.

ADVANCED
1 Big O kiss

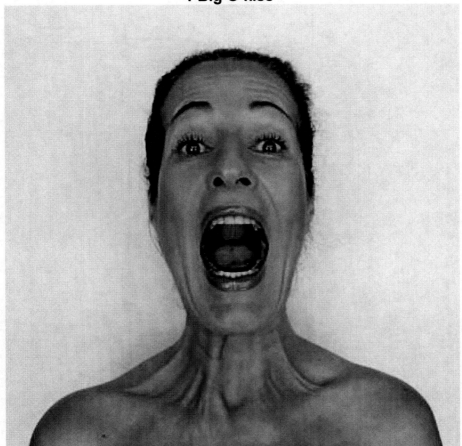

TARGET Warm up - whole face

1. Open your mouth as wide as you can
2. Raise your eyebrows (pulling everything back)
3. Pause for a moment
4. Slowly bring your lips in to form a kiss with your eyebrows into a slight frown
5. Pause for a moment

- Repeat continuously for 20 repetitions

ADVANCED
2 Eyebrow lifts

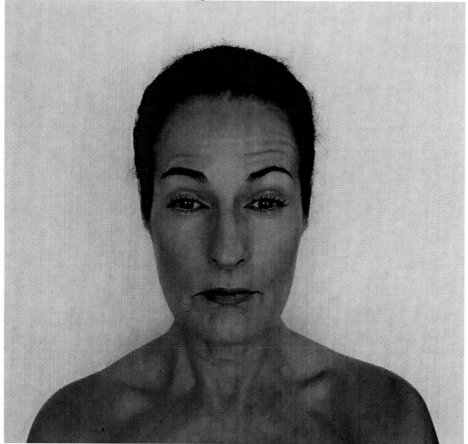

TARGET Brow, eyebrows & upper eyelid

1. Smile gently and hold
2. Lift your eyebrows as high as possible and pause for a couple of seconds
3. Relax

- Repeat approximately 30 times
- Total 1 minute

Note:
Feel as if, you are raising and lowering your eyebrows slowly.

ADVANCED
3 Face-lift

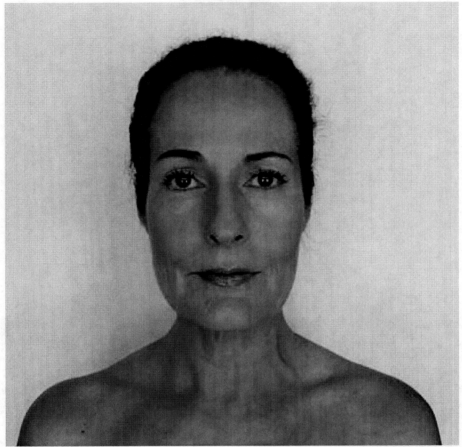

TARGET Whole face, especially forehead and cheekbones

1. With eyes open (easier) or shut
2. Lift eyebrows
3. Contract muscle of scalp and temples, lifting you eyebrows up and back to connect with the back of the neck.
- Hold for I minute
- Repeat twice (i.e. for a total of 3 times)

Note:
Feel the whole face pull taut, up and back. Imagine that your whole skull is being tightened, lifted and pulled back.
Tip: Ensure that the sides of your mouth are level with the corners slightly turning up. **DO NOT FROWN**

ADVANCED
4 Eye pulls

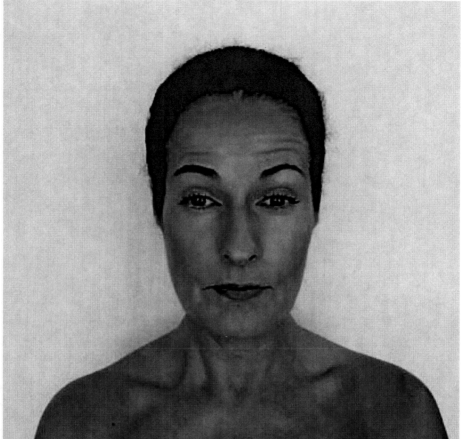

TARGET All around the eyes, both corners, plus under eyelids

1. Begin with eyes shut firmly
2. Raise the eyebrows
3. Try to open your eyes very slowly, for a count of approximately 20 seconds
4. When almost fully open, hold for a count of 10
5. Relax

• Repeat

Note:
This is a difficult exercise to master but you will feel those bags lifting.

ADVANCED
5 Clocks (closed)

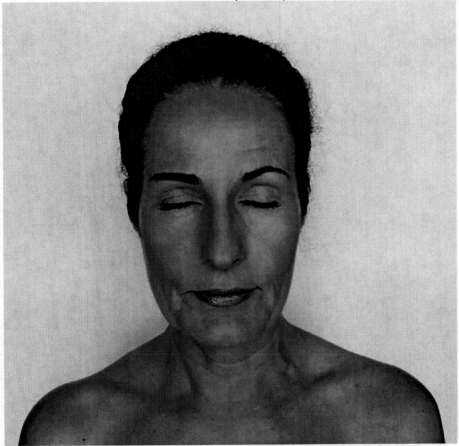

TARGET Sides of eyes

1. Lift your eyes up and rotate slowly clockwise for 3 revolutions
2. Repeat anticlockwise

Note:
Each revolution should take about 10 seconds. Extend your glance fully in each direction.

ADVANCED
6 Bag lifts

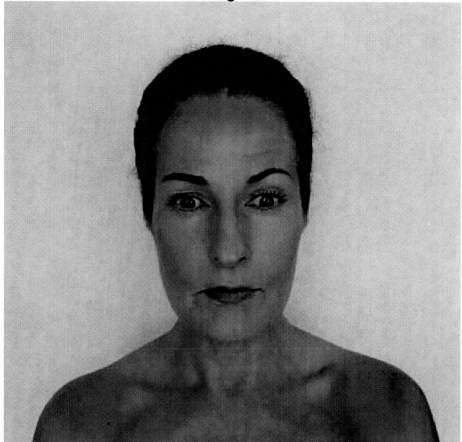

TARGET Sides of eyes

1. Raise eyebrows slightly
2. With eyes open, lift the under eye area as high as possible, pause hold for a count of 5
3. Lower under eyelid
4. Raise and repeat lifting up pause, down

- Repeat 10 times

ADVANCED
7 Bunny noses

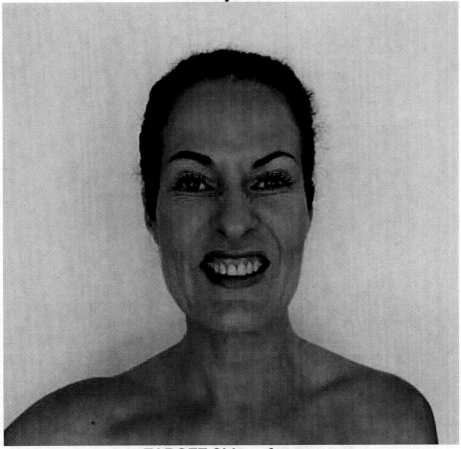

TARGET Sides of nose

1. Open your mouth slightly and crinkle your nose
2. Slowly make forward circular motions, up forwards, down and around with the tip of your nose and top lip

• Repeat 20 times in one direction and then reverse
  Continue doing this for approximately 1 minute

ADVANCED
8 In and out kisses

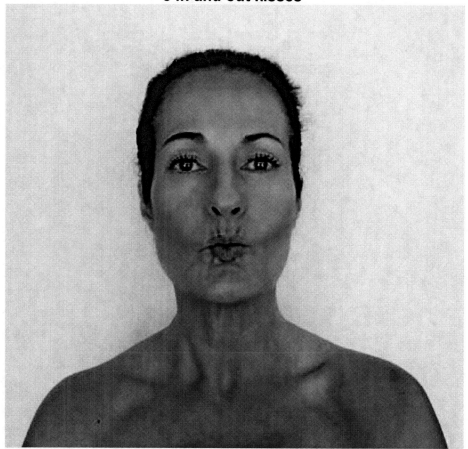

TARGET Sides of nose and cheeks

1. With closed lips, slowly smile broadly to the earlobes
2. Pause for a couple of second
3. Slowly move lips forward into a kiss
4. Pause, for a couple of seconds, keep the tension repeat continuously

- Lift eyebrows (if you want an extra pull)
- Repeat continuously for about 1 minute

Note:
Try to ensure that the corners of the mouth are upright.

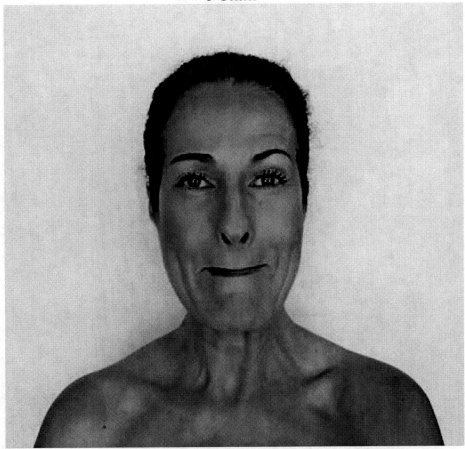

TARGET Cheeks, under eye area & eyebrows

1. Pull top lip over teeth
2. Push bottom jaw forward and pull bottom lip over teeth
3. Pull up sides of nose, cheeks
4. Lift eyebrows (if you want an extra pull)

- Hold continuously for approximately 1 minute

Note:
This is difficult and may take you a while to master, start with holding for less time and work up to one minute.

ADVANCED
10 Three smiles

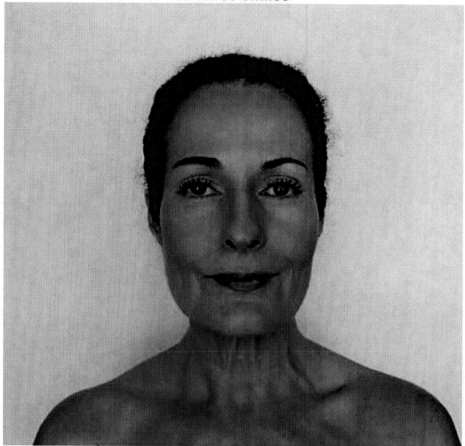

TARGET Cheeks & jowls

1. Lips together smile horizontally, hold for a count of 10
2. Lips together smile more towards the earlobes, hold 10 count
3. Lips together make a huge smile temples, count to 10
4. Lips together smile towards earlobes, hold count to 10

- Keeping the tension repeat

Note:
This is difficult to master. It is like smiling up once, twice, three times then letting go of the smile once, twice and starting up again.

ADVANCED
11 Jaw lifts

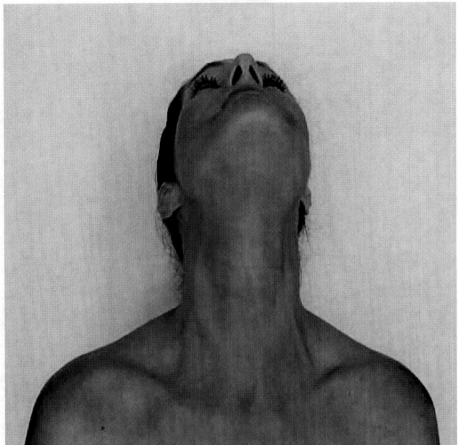

TARGET Neck & chin

1. With mouth closed thrust your lower jaw forwards
2. Make a wide grin curling the lips and corner of the mouth up
3. Extend your neck, relax shoulders and gently tilt your head back
4. With your head resting backwards thrust your chin towards the ceiling
5. Pause for a moment
6. Repeat 10 times in succession
7. Relax
8. Bring head forward

• Repeat

ADVANCED
12 Chin dimples

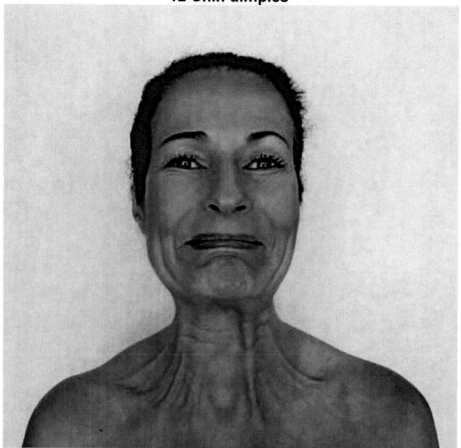

TARGET Chin & neck

1. Close your mouth and clench your teeth
2. Pull the corners of your mouth down, your neck muscles should stand out
3. Force the corners of your mouth upwards, this should make divots in your chin
4. Hold for a count of 30

• Repeat

Note:
This is very difficult, do not strain too much. If you find it too difficult do not repeat.

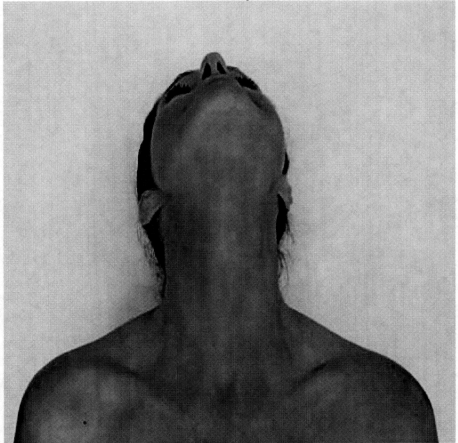

TARGET Chin & neck

1. Sit upright , relax your shoulders , extend your neck and gently drop the head backwards
2. Look at the ceiling while keeping your lips closed and relaxed
3. Open your mouth and bring your lower jaw forward and upward trying to get your lower teeth to cover your top teeth.
4. Hold for a count of 10
5. Relax, bring head gently towards

- Repeat 3 times

Note:
This is hard exercise, use extreme caution.

ADVANCED
14 Neck flex

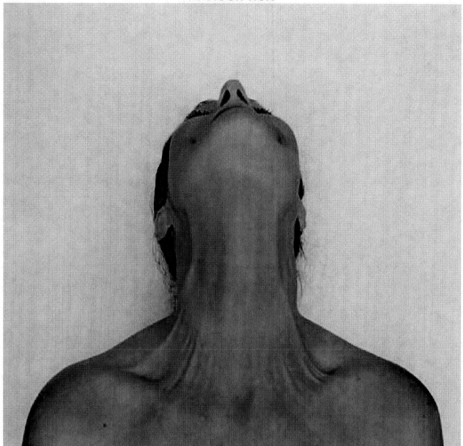

TARGET Neck

1. Clench your teeth and spread your bottom lip,(your neck muscles will flex)
2. Keeping the tension, extend your neck, relax your shoulders and gently drop your head backwards to rest on your shoulders
3. Lift and lower your head 5 times in succession
4. Relax the tension and raise your head to an upright position

• Repeat

Note:
This is a very hard neck muscle exercise, be careful

ADVANCED
15 Ears relaxation

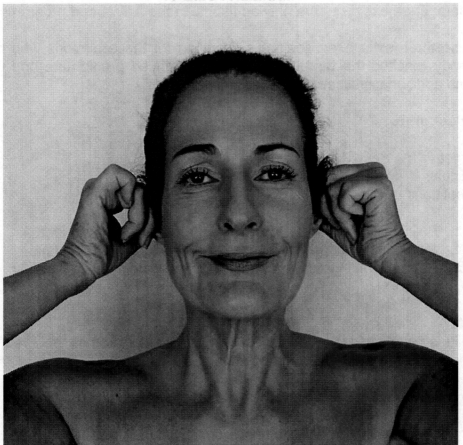

TARGET Ears & jowls

1. Pinch your earlobes and massage between fingers moving up the back of the ear coming all the way to the front
2. Put your index finger in your ear hole and gently rotate your finger to massage inner ear whilst your thumb gently massages the back of the outer ear

Extra Exercises

(Note: Extra exercises are only additional to the **Advanced** programme)

These three extra exercises were designed for those persons who have already reached the target level of the Advanced programme and want some additional choices to attack a problem area.

Widest grins

Target	Upper cheeks
Difficulty	Very hard
Repetitions	30

1. Pull your widest smile, showing your teeth and crow's feet
2. Simultaneously raise eyebrows and cheeks, pause, release
3. Repeat continuously (maintaining the widest smile), slowly, with control

Note:
Smile is maintained, nose wrinkles as the opposite force as the eyebrows and cheeks are worked up and down.

Under eye lifts

Target	Under eye bags
Difficulty	Very hard
Hold	60 seconds

1. Raise the eyebrows
2. Lift the area under the eye, until the lower eyelid is horizontally across the eye pupil
3. Hold for I minute

Side chin thrust

Target	Jowls chin and neck
Difficulty	Very hard
Hold	10 counts
Repetitions	3 to each side

1. Extend your neck
2. Gently drop your head backwards
3. Push jaw forwards
4. Move jaw to the left and hold, for a count of ten. Automatically the left corner of your mouth should rise up to the outer corner of your eye
5. Move jaw to the right and hold, for a count of ten. Automatically the right corner of your mouth should rise up to the outer corner of your eye

Note:
To increase the pull push your lips forwards.

Chapter 11

Final Words

Maintaining a youthful lifestyle

Your lifestyle habits can slow down, if not reverse the normal ageing process thus making you appear more youthful. Eating healthy foods and exercise will make your body healthier in turn make you feel and look healthier. This change will also be reflected in the appearance of your skin. You will glow from the inside out. What have you got to lose, only wrinkles!

Food nutrition

This is the single most important thing you can do for yourself, your body and your skin. Diet is so important, pack it full of goodness. Remember your skin grows from the inside out. However, this is not a book on nutrition; I have just included a few pointers to encourage you towards a healthy diet.

These are my top tips for good balanced diet:

- Enjoy eating food
- Eat a variety of different foods
- Eat the correct amount to maintain a healthy weight (not skin and bones)
- Eat plenty of fruit and vegetables
- Eat plenty of foods rich in starch and fibre
- Reduce fat and sugary goods
- Drink alcohol in moderation

Eat a balanced diet; that does not mean eating the same size portions of each food but rather implies to include many foods within your diet but in the right proportions for each food group.

A healthy balanced diet contains a variety of foods including plenty of fruit and vegetables, plenty of starchy foods such as wholegrain bread, pasta and rice, some protein-rich foods such as meat, fish, eggs and lentils and some dairy foods. It should also be low in fat (especially saturated fat), salt and sugar.

A healthy diet is one that helps maintain or improve health. It is important for the prevention of many chronic health risks such as: obesity, heart disease, diabetes, and cancer.

A healthy diet involves consuming appropriate amounts of all nutrients, and an adequate amount of water. Nutrients can be obtained from many different foods, so there are a wide variety of diets that may be considered healthy diets.

5-A-DAY

The abandoned American phrase was coined by the British government to educate "the youth of today" to eat fruit and vegetables. Walk into any British supermarket and you will see "1 portion" in the chilled (deli) section. The supermarkets jumped on the bandwagon and introduced these small portions for children's lunchboxes, a packed lunch that they take to school. Examples of which are cut up applies, carrots, grapes, all of which helps the busy mum in the morning get the children off to school.

At all costs try to eat '5 a day', that is five portions of fruit and vegetables a day is essential. This will do you more good than anything else; you will glow from the inside out. That is how your body works, your body needs energy from good nutrition and as far as **Fitface** is concerned, how the skin grows and facial muscles develop.

Choose from fresh, frozen, canned, dried or juiced, anything is better than nothing but don't cheat to such an extent as to eat tinned fruit in syrup or put too much cream and sugar on a fruit salad that the bad outweighs the good!

Be sensible, don't be silly by eating not only your '5 a day' but also stuffing yourself full of sweets, chocolates and fatty fast foods. One just eliminates the other! Just try to make a lifestyle change to a healthy eating pattern. Processed foods not only lose most of its nutrition by all the additives of flavorings, fats, colours and processing but also preservation.

Green supplements are just that, there to supplement your diet, they do help but they are not the real thing, they are not designed to replace 'real food'. Eat your greens, enjoy them. Yes, I know they take a long time to prepare but you can cheat a little with things like for example frozen peas.

Fruit

Almost nothing is better for you; within oranges, lemons, grapefruits, pineapples, mangos, papayas, peaches, nectarines etc you can almost see the sunshine in every piece, that's natural energy! There are no fillers, no additives, just goodness. What's more they taste great!

Eat it raw

Try eating fruit and vegetables raw whenever you can, it's quicker and easier and best of all, it's better for you. Fruit and vegetables have lost many of their essential nutrients in the transportation and storage before they even reach you. Then, if you cook them, even more essential vitamins are lost. So, just try 'eating raw' one day a week. Even the pressure of cutting and chopping looses nutrients!

Starchy foods containing carbohydrates

The food group that includes such foods as: bread, oats, maize, other cereals, cornmeal, pasta, yams, potatoes and rice. (Note: I didn't include biscuits, cakes, pastries, potato crisps, pretzels, bagels or muffins)! Contrary to popular belief these foods are not fattening in moderation; it is what we put with them that makes them fattening i.e. by adding fats and rich sauces. Try to eat wholegrain, wholemeal or high fibre versions of carbohydrates whenever, and wherever possible. This is because they contain more fibre which is advantageous because;

- Soluble fibre has been shown to lower cholesterol levels
- Prevents constipation
- Helps protect against bowel problems
- Helps control the appetite by making you feel fuller longer
- Slower release of sustained energy

Avoid processed foods

You know this is sound advice. You only have to look at the colour or lack of it in most processed foods; they are dull, not like when you cut open fresh fruit.

You don't have time so you just grab something or stop at a takeaway? Try to enjoy cooking, maybe get some new books, recipes. Have a go. Eating real food will energise you and make you and your skin glow.

Quorn

However of course we all need processed foods. I am a vegetarian and could not live, or rather, would prefer not to do without Quorn. I think it is a fantastic product, far better than soy products and I can't stand tofu, it is so tasteless. Personally I especially like the ground beef Quorn for making spaghetti bolognaise the Quorn chicken bits for stir-fry's and deli slices. In England and Europe generally they have a large selection of these products, there I like the chicken slices for sandwiches and picnics – English weather permitting!

Vitamin pills, powdered protein, compounds and supplements

They must not be taken to replace food, which is why most of the time they are called a supplement, i.e. **they add to an already good balanced diet**. They should not be used to replace food, although they can be an excellent source of addition nutrition or as a substitute occasionally when the real thing is not available.

I am especially concerned by people who habitually combine these artificially reproduced supplements in the belief that they are giving their bodies a very healthy diet containing all the trace elements, minerals and vitamins required for proper nutrition. My primary worry is that the body may not be able to correctly absorb the chemicals within these supplements as the natural digestive process is extremely complex. Therefore these people who eat hardly anything and rely on protein drinks, vitamin pills and supplements are surely not getting what nature intended in the way of real nutrition?

Of increasing unease to me, is the American obsession with protein powders. These generally taste revolting but somehow have become very popular, the result of overzealous pyramid marketing by protein powder suppliers cashing in on the insecurities of others. Protein can be found naturally easily and less expensively, the body only needs a small amount daily.

However, I would agree that food is not what it used to be because of the lack of nutrition in the soil due to intensive farming and consequently the lack of trace elements, vitamins and minerals in our food. For example in the last 50 years runner beans have lost 10% of its copper, broccoli 75% of its calcium, watercress 90% of its copper, steak 55% of its iron and cheddar cheese 38% of its magnesium. Levels of other important minerals including magnesium, iron phosphorous and potassium have also plummeted. Is it any wonder we need supplements, but buyer beware, some are better than others.

My daughter had "tests" and told me that being a vegetarian like myself she lacked Vitamin B-12, so I have just started taking it.

Metabolism

Metabolism is a hugely complex subject. The body can manufacture many of the nutrients it needs but this manufacturing must draw on a vast array of nutrients which can only be obtained from the diet. However, nowadays many nutrients are missing from the soil that our food is grown in. Therefore eating correctly and taking a supplement maybe necessary, unless you grow your own in organically enriched soil.

Weight control

The thyroid regulates the burning of calories and affects every cell in the body, regulating cell metabolism like a thermostat. Low function doesn't produce enough active hormones, so the system becomes inert. Weight tends to go up as the thyroid function goes down and vice versa. Although iodine is often thought to be the critical factor, equally the balance of micronutrients involved in the delicate metabolic processes involved in feeding the thyroid are all important.

Weight loss

Weight loss without proper detoxification leads to environmental pollutants that are stored in body fat cells being released into the blood stream. As blood levels rise, levels of essential thyroid hormones (necessary to maintain efficient metabolism fall dramatically - adaptive thermogenisis). A concomitant reduction in muscle oxidative enzymes (which determine how efficiently the muscles use energy), results in energy being stored as fat, creating a vicious cycle – weight loss/rising blood contaminations/loss of oxidative enzymes/increase in fat. Detoxification is needed.

Liquids

Water

It is no secret that the body is over 70% water and therefore we need it to survive. Drink plenty of water, enjoy it, try different varieties, experiment, have fun. Somewhere I read that 64 ounces of water per day is recommended, I agree that sounds like a lot! 8 x 8oz glasses sound more reasonable but it is the same! Put another way that's 4 pints.

I am not sure that I am convinced about water sold in plastic bottles. I read somewhere, that if the plastic bottle gets warm, harmful chemicals and dioxins can be released from the plastic and can leak into the water. Dioxin Carcinogens cause cancer, I know what doesn't? But if I have taken a sip of water from my drinking bottle and it has been left in the sun it tastes peculiar. Therefore what about here and throughout the world when it is being transported by road in tarpaulin covered trucks (lorries) sometimes for days in the blazing heat. Surely, if nothing else this degrades the product?

Alcohol

Is fine in moderation but that's it! Red wine is reputed to be positively good for you; well that is a glass (not mega sized) or perhaps two a day. One of the worst things about alcohol is the dehydrating effect it has on the body and therefore the skin bur also increasing your cholesterol levels! Unbelievable but true. I have also heard/read that liver damage from drinking too much alcohol can be seen on the sides at the top of the nose as blue coloration. Sadly it looks like I have fallen victim, have you?

Sodas, carbonated (fizzy) or energy drinks

We all know they are no good for you but oh they are tempting. Try to wean yourself off them your skin will look better for it.

Salt

Salt is an acquired taste. This means that, while the foods you eat will taste bland when you first cut back on salt, soon your taste buds will adapt and you won't even notice the difference. In fact, the foods you eat will probably taste better than ever when you stop dulling your senses with so much salt. You can look better and add years to your life by cutting back on salt. (Taken from McKinley Health Centre, University of Illinois, citing R. L. Duyff, American Dietetic Association's Complete Food and Nutrition Guide, 1998).

Salt replacements just add potassium to compensate for the taste, try something new like a seaweed compound, preferably made from Wrack or Dulse seaweed. I try to use natural sea salt; it is expensive but tastes great. But hey if I run out, I use the regular stuff, life is too short.

Personally I highly recommend Himalayan Salt, maybe it is just hype but it sounds convincing and best of all tastes great. Yes it is expensive; you get what you pay for!

Himalayan Salt

Himalayan salt contains all the minerals and trace elements of which our bodies are made. Natural salt is crucial for maintaining vital functions in the body. Himalayan salt has no preservatives or additives. Doctors and alternative therapists agree that Himalayan salt is the cleanest salt available on the planet to deliver remarkable health benefits. Himalayan crystal salt is pristine and natural. It consists of the most perfect geometric structure possible in rock crystals, the result of millions of years of compression under the Earth's surface. It has the precise mesh with our body's inner workings because Himalayan salt contains an almost identical set of elements to those found inside the human body, 84 of the possible 92 trace minerals, in the same proportion as naturally exists in our blood.

Exercise

I need not ramble on here about the merit of exercise, there has been already enough written on the subject, we all know it's great for you, this book is about a specific type of exercise. Any type of exercise: be it running, swimming, gardening, walking the dog or even a mammoth shopping trip will not only make you look better but also you'll feel better both mentally and physically.

Skincare

Personally I believe in keeping to a simple routine. The skin is made to be self cleaning, look how clean animals are. The skin is an important natural barrier, the function of which is to keep moisture in and outside invaders out. We are obsessed with keeping the skin squeaky clean which is not necessarily the best thing for it. Overzealous toning and too much vigorous exfoliation (in the hope of revealing newer brighter skin underneath) can strip away the skins vital natural protection. There was recently a study made of the 'cleanliness' of unwashed skin and bacterially there was no significant difference with unwashed skin after 3 weeks!

According to the many of beauty experts one of the biggest challenges facing our complexions today isn't pollution or sun damage – its cosmetic overload. By mid-life, the average American woman is using between fifteen to twenty products on her skin in a typical day. All you really need at most is a good cleanser and moisturiser that can be used both day and night.

The manufacturers of all those expensive creams would not approve of my routine. I use nothing but water to wash my face followed by a simple moisturizing cream (I used to use all sorts of lotions and potions). My philosophy is that if the Queen, her majesty, Queen Elizabeth 2nd of the United Kingdom cannot look younger (with all her money and advisors) being the world's most public figure, then it stands to reason that the rest of us have little chance with creams alone. Furthermore I understand that the large molecules of many of these skin preparations cannot penetrate into the pores of the skin, they simply don't fit in and it is really is as simple as that; at best they smell nice and feel good but many just glide over the surface. Most hydrate the skin which can only be a good thing and many also protect it from the sun's harmful rays. So by all means do use one, but it is not necessary to pay a fortune. If you like the bottle on your dressing table fair enough however, wouldn't the feel good factor of giving the savings to your charity of choice give you more of an emotional *lift*?

Today there are many new creams on the market with all sorts of ingredients that are suppose to make you look younger. Well I don't know? I have read the research, much of which seems convincing and after all there is progress, so if it makes you feel good and you think you look better go for it, what harm can it do? Well, actually some can, unfortunately and often unwittingly some products strip away the skin's acid mantel (a thin coating of oil and perspiration that helps protect you from infections and bacteria). Be cautious of harsh soaps or toners which can disrupt your skin's natural balance of acidity and salinity (called PH balance). Also be aware that too much moisturiser may not be a good thing as the barrier is supposed to be permeable allowing bad toxins to evaporate through the surface.

If and when I wear foundation/make up or eye shadow I gently remove the majority of the excess with E45 lotion or similar on a cotton pad. I do not pull and stretch the skin (or rub for all I am worth) or indeed take off every scrap. Around the eyes I use cotton swabs (buds); I do not pull and stretch but dab. I have never taken off my mascara, it just comes off naturally (most especially after I have washed my hair) and I separate my wet eyelashes with an old dry brush mascara brush, thus unclogging and removing any residue. However, almost every morning I remove the smudged dark "bits" under my eyes with a cotton swab (bud) dipped in good non greasy E45 (a cheap, over the counter dermatological moisturizing lotion that is perfume free and hypoallergenic). Sadly it's not FDA approved and is only available in the UK so Mummie sends it to me.

I wasn't going to mention this because it sounds weird but.... Sometimes I come in late at night, say after a party and my make-up feels all glued to my skin so I used *wipes* that I found at the "Dollar Store" (pound shop). I first tried specifically designed make-up remover wipes but found them too harsh. I then moved on to baby wipes and again found them too astringent. Liking "wipes" for the ease of use I progressed to "Intimate Wipes" and thought and still think they are great. I told my friend about them and she, (unlike me) read the package. It says "Alcohol and Paraben Free Formula"and is stamped with Aloe Vera logo. The reverse says "The high PH value of regular soaps may change the PH balance of your genital area leaving your skin weak against irritations and infections. However, Lucky super soft intimate wipes are harmonious with the natural PH value of your body." Ah ha, that's why I like them!

I don't use face packs, masks, scrubs, or astringents, night creams, anti-ageing creams, wrinkle creams or anything exotic. I have in the past but, so much has been written about how they don't work I guess it's finally

221

sunk in as a flagrant waste of money. Once again I repeat what my mother would say of the Queen, "She can afford to use anything in the world she wants and has numerous advisors to recommend her all the best products on earth but at the end of the day she still looks like an old lady," so too would all the celebrities - without needles or the knife. Ageing is a natural process, embrace it, just be the best you can be!

Spas

I covered spas earlier in the book as they have changed drastically from being places of tranquility where natural beauty treatments and healing therapies were offered to, in some instances, what can only be described as outpatient's centres. Traditional spas seem to make everyone feel wonderful. Personally I feel a little silly and shy but that could be because I am British. I have yet to get into them and go with the flow. They seem to work wonders for everyone, concentrating the mind body and soul not to mention hydrating and replenishing the skin, therefore if you enjoy it, feel relaxed and can afford them, go ahead if it makes you feel good, it will do you good.

Bathing

Fragrance manufacturers don't like me either, too much is made of "smellies" and I find it especially odd since we are fundamentally using all these 'perfumed' products to be more attractive towards the opposite sex, however men actually prefer the smell of pheromones! Your natural body odour; therefore I rarely use anything in baths or showers and especially no harsh detergents. Besides they either seem to leave a residue on me, or in the bath, therefore I can only imagine they clog or dry the skin. Of course they do smell nice to use and occasionally I will have a dash of something non-drying in a bath for the feel good relaxing feeling and obviously I shower with soap or a simple shower gel.

Hair washing

I am not fanatical about washing my hair, it is not squeaky clean, and I wash and blow dry when I'm going out otherwise I just let it be. When it gets tangled, about every third day, I jump under the shower and run only conditioner through it, it's the only way I can get a brush, (let alone comb) through it. I think that way, when I want it to look nice my hair has had some chance to recover from the torture of constant washing and drying and hopefully some of the natural oils have returned. I nearly always cut and dye my hair myself. There is no way I could afford to keep up with the maintenance payments of a hair salon! I do admit it never looks even close to as good as the hair dresser but hey ho, there is more to life!

Hair brushing

For about the last few years I have begun to copy my mother in her "hair brushing routine". She vigorously brushes her hair daily or rather massages her scalp. I cannot always get through my hair, so I do what I can; brushing at the edges with a *thing* I bought in "Sally's" (hair salon supply store open to the public in the USA). I think it is for Afro-Caribbean type hair. It is a plastic oval about 3 inches across by 2 inches with lots of short half inch spikes.

No I haven't lost the plot; I feel certain that it has improved the growth and quality of my hair, the trade off is that there's more breakage and split ends. Maybe it is also good to exercise to get the blood flowing to the whole head as opposed to just the face, it must improve circulation i.e. nutrition being brought to the hair follicles. Well it's now part of my routine and I have thick long hair whereas some of my friends are becoming increasingly bald, so maybe there's something in it?

Stress

Is the number one killer and it shows on the face. Just try to relax which is easier said than done. Try to take yourself to a less stressful scene and think of the bigger picture. Is 'it' that important in the context of one's whole life? Do not make mountains out of mole hills and remember other people have lives to live and their problems, stresses and strains are just as real as yours!

Unwind, all work and no play, is not good for anyone.

Sleep

It is a myth that one requires eight hours; new research shows that 7 hours is ample. If you find sleeping a problem get up and do something you don't want to do! Cleaning a window, a mirror, checking your bank statement, tidying the bits and pieces in a drawer, choose anything so long as it's boring. That way you will be training yourself that waking up and not dropping off is not much fun. You must not train yourself to be rewarded for example with a cup of hot chocolate and a good book or guess what, you will wake up and have some more fun!

Sleep is when the body repairs and rebuilds itself and especially those all important muscles, collagen and elastin. So you are warned. If you sleep better you will look better and it's free.

There is a school of thought that you should lie on your back so as not to form wrinkles. Well I'm not so sure about that. I tend to sleep on my face! So I thought a little more about the subject. When I lay on my stomach, my relaxed facial skin hangs down from my muscles and bones and is flattered on the bed. As opposed to if I were laying the other way around, my skin would be draped over my face sinking into any relaxed pockets. This could be an interesting medical experiment!

Sun

Surely all the messages have gotten through without me having to write about the number one ageing effect caused by over exposure to ultraviolet light i.e. sun damaged. If you must sunbathe then do so with heavy sun cream protection when the sun is lower in the sky for a short amount of time. Alternatively cover up completely and use a fake tan on your face. I know it's difficult I too love sunbathing for short periods.

It's hard to refrain from doing something you like; so if you are a sun worshiper, wear sunscreen and at least try to cut down your sun exposure a little.

Central heating

If you live in a cold climate and have the central heating on almost 24/7 for the winter months do ensure that you sleep in a well ventilated room and place a bowl of water in the room to prevent the air becoming too drying. Try it; you will be surprised how much will evaporates!

Air conditioning

If you live in a hot country air conditioning is not particularly kind to the face either, it takes the humidity out of the air, thus robbing the skin it of its natural hydration. Make up for the body being dehydrated by drinking a little more water and do try turning the AC down a notch or two!

Smoking

Once again I should not have to mention how socially unacceptable it is and repeat the media/advertising messages that it is bad for the skin, smoking is very ageing, therefore don't. I should know I was almost yellow from the nicotine before I quit.

Try all the methods to quit available, one of them may work? Personally I've found that the nicotine replacement supplements helped me, in fact I got to the stage where I preferred the gum or pills to the real thing - cigarettes). Whatever works for you, just keep trying to quit – never give up on trying quitting. My American friend swears by Chantix, a pill taken once daily.

Lose 10 lbs instantly

On the subject of being all you can be, I just felt that I could add this funny anecdote that I was sent over the internet.

If you are no more than 10lbs overweight, currently I probably am at 130lbs, (and I do stress currently – in the hopes that my weight will miraculously go down) 5' 6" (but I tell everyone 5' 7" hey maybe I can get back there with yoga) it's all muscle, they say, yeah sure. Actually I have been working out and doing tons of yoga this year so I reckon I am back to 5' 7" – and I am down to 128.3 lbs, I digress.

The instant 10lbs weight loss story

Simply mimic who you wanted to be in the mirror. Most of us stand there and play with our images, i.e. we suck in our stomachs (lose an easy 5lbs), stretch taller (got to be worth 3lb's) stick out our boobs (a loss of 2lb's in terms of 'the line') clench and protrude buttocks/bottom (let's face it if you are over 45 that alone is worth 5lbs - but shall we say 3lbs) a total loss of 13lbs. To complete the instant remake add a smile, think happy thoughts, love the world and "Bobs your uncle", you are set to "rock n' roll" and look 10lbs lighter!

Endorsements for facial exercise programmes

There are tons and tons and tons of materials available hailing the positive effects of exercising however, the information on facial exercising is scant. This I find odd as I cannot possibly understand why, if exercising is considered so good for the body, that it is not regarded as the same for the face? It is preposterous! It is as if the cells, blood and tissue of the face are different from the rest of the body. **Is it not in fact more important to exercise the face?** If only, because; the brain is the most vital of all organs! It controls the rest of the body, and is housed in the skull directly behind the face. Surely, increasing blood flow to the brain, thereby sending more nutrients and oxygen there, can only be a good thing? Doesn't that imply that the brain should work more efficiently? Is that not the reason that all sorts of vitamen supplements to increase brain activity such as cognitive thinking are sold?

The head is where all the sense organs are located. Unquestionably we all need:
- good eyesight
- good hearing
- a good sense of smell
- a good sense of taste
- and the skin's sense of nerve sensibility to pressure (touch), temperature, etc

Therefore, must I not conclude, (as a reasonably intelligent human being) that performing facial exercises which stimulates an increased supply of oxygen and nutrients to the head/face/brain are beneficial to the brain? The opposite/alternative argument is in my opinion "daft!"

Professor's endorsements – Indiana.

Sept 2009. **Professor Stuart Warden**, Director of Physical Therapy Research at Indiana University, informed the New York Times last week that "The stresses of exercise activate a particular molecular pathway that increases collagen, which leads to stronger connective tissues in the dermis, and thus, fewer wrinkles and younger-looking skin."

Dr. R. Ray – Washington, DC.

"Regarding face exercises, I completely agree that a lot can be done to change the structural appearance of the face through muscular exercise not just in the context of ageing, but as an alternative to some of the plastic surgery that has been getting more popular. Actually, I imagine it would produce a more psychologically comfortable outcome, since I imagine people would feel the same sense of ownership, that it is still their face, rather than a face that has been surgically engineered."

Famous American TV physician's endorsements:

1. **Dr. Oz** wrote in the book, he mentioned on his show that a Japanese study that may give credence to the idea that facial exercises work.

2. Dermatologist, **Dr. Nicholas Perricone**, shares Dr. Oz's viewpoint regarding facial exercises. On his Blog Page, MD Perricone, states that, "If your skin has already begun to lose its tone and elasticity, natural face-lift options are available." Dr. Perricone states that, in fact, there are several ways to firm up your skin and that some of the best ways involve natural remedies such as proper diet and nutrition, taking supplements and getting plenty of exercise.

   He stated that, "Exercise is one of the most important practises to maintain for firming your skin. Exercise will help circulation which ultimately results in skin remaining firm and toned." Dr. Perricone sums it up succinctly by stating, "Simple facial exercises are great for tightening the skin of the face."

   I have read much of what Dr Perricone says in his books including "The Wrinkle Cure and 7 secrets to Beauty, Health and Longevity." I have seen Dr. Oz's TV show and it reaches to the heart of America.

One of Beverly Hills most famous plastic surgeons and a TV personality.

When initially researching this book, I wrote to this plastic surgeon (and thousands of other surgeons) and asked them for their opinion on facial exercises.

My original letter to him and many other plastic/cosmetic surgeons:

Dear Dr....
Facial Exercise Research

Do you or do you not (pre or post surgery) support (or recommend) facial exercises as a preventative or alternative to face lifts/eye, brow, forehead surgical procedures? Your help would be most appreciated.
Thanking you in advance for your co-operation. Any comments that you would be so kind as to supply, would of course, remain strictly confidential.

Charlotte Hamilton

This very famous surgeon graciously replied:
"I do support the use of facial exercises. They work! However, I do many face-lifts when the age has gone past the ability of exercises to make the difference."

Other eminent USA physicians:

Mark Berman, M.D.

Past President of the California Academy of Cosmetic Surgeons. Santa Monica, CA, stated:

"I've seen the results and they're really quite impressive."

"Actually if you think about it, this makes sense medically. After all, when you exercise your body, you're going to tone and tighten the muscles in your body. So why not apply the same principles to your face."

The Board of Trustees of the American Academy of Cosmetic Surgery has approved the nomination of Dr. Berman for President 2010 (President - Elect 2009). Dr. Berman named to "Super Doctors List" by Los Angeles Magazine, December 2009 and January 2010.

Margret Olsen, MD Los Angeles, CA

"Many people want to improve their appearance but do not want to have to go through surgery. We are finding that facial exercises can really make a difference in toning muscles and making them stronger. Such as people with droopy necks."

Physicians generally

In Europe many physicians prescribe specific facial exercise programmes post cosmetic surgery but that is surely like bolting the door after the horse has left the stable?

There are many physicians that have publically endorsed facial exercise for their own sake. Please refer to the Internet for their names.

China – the next Superpower

It is mandatory for all Chinese school children to twice daily, in the classroom to perform facial exercises to improve their eyesight. Unfortunately these are not "hands free". But obviously the Chinese government believes they work or they would not take the measure to enforce billions of Chinese to improve their health.

Nintendo

I have already covered the greatest endorsement that facial exercises could ever have i.e. that of Nintendo DS and Wii publishers under Touch aka "Facening" launched in Japan in October 2006. Obviously, the multimillion dollar technological giant must have spent millions (if not billions of dollars) in research and development together with extensive health and safety checks before so publically acknowledging that facial exercises are fun, beneficial and safe.

Face Training on DSi or DSi XL was launched in September 2010 on primetime British TV, whether or not the product will reach the USA remains to be seen. Perhaps I am being too cynical? But with the financial clout behind the medical profession, coupled with the rapidly growing public acceptability of cosmetic procedures I seriously doubt it!

My personal endorsements

Originally I had intended to make the website and the **Fitface toning** guide very personal; being all about me, showing various photographs of myself ending with current ones (well there are a few **see Chapter 3**) to show that even at my age (54) I do not have any of the first (severe) signs of ageing in the commonly advertised A zone which are:

- **Nasolabial folds**

The deep folds that begin at the sides of the nose and run down to beyond the corners of the mouth. This is one of the first signs of ageing although younger people with prominent fatty cheek pads may also have prominent nasolabial folds

- **Frown lines**
  Vertical lines, also called glabellar lines that appear between the eyebrows
- **Wrinkles**
  Across the top of the nose

Additionally my horizontal forehead lines or worry lines as they are commonly called are only a little visible.

I was also going to include a sworn testimonial from a prominent surgeon who had examined me to check that I have never had any **facial surgery or fillers of any kind**, ever. However, I thought that it was going over the top. Although I am 100% open to any examination and challenge anyone to find anything.

The rest of the endorsements and content of **Fitface toning** was going to be stories and testimonials from various friends and clients showing the normal before and after photos of all those people that I have helped over the years. However, I felt that this could be misinterpreted and unfair as everyone will benefit from **Fitface toning**. Each person's face is only one of a kind, every one of us will progress through the **Fitface** training at different rates and the many changes to appearance will all be at varying degrees. So I wanted **Fitface toning** to be all about you, about your **Fitface toning**. Not about me, or anyone else's before and after shots but yours. It is all about you, the unique person that you are and how you look and feel. If everyone compares themselves with each other then the message is lost. There is no competition. It is about being the best you can be. **Fitface toning** was designed to naturally enhance your own unique beauty.

Last word

Hopefully you will have had the self discipline and strength of character to stick to the **Fitface toning** routine for the first three months and therefore improvements in your facial tone have begun to show.

When this happens, tell the world. Tell everyone you know; your friends, your associates, your colleagues and most especially your doctor. This way, perhaps the word will spread about **Fitface toning** facial exercises, and the world can put away the desire for unnecessary cosmetic surgery and live in the light of being who they are not what someone, at a fashion trend magazine thinks you were meant to be.

Information

References

Major sources of general information

Throughout the writing of **Fitface** I have sourced a massive amount of information from books, the internet and consulted with many surgeons.

My primary source of information was the internet and therefore I have included only some of the more relevant websites surrounding each issue and a little specific source information.

There were hundreds and hundreds of hours spent in many libraries throughout England and the United States of America reading medical reference books for example, **Cosmetic and Reconstructive Surgery Sourcebook - Health Reference Series**. Those books that I could take home I did. Some I purchased like the "**Winkle Cure**" and "**Seven Secrets to Beauty, Health and Longevity**" Nicholas Perricone M.D and "**Straight talk about cosmetic surgery**" Arthur W. Perry (a private practice cosmetic surgeon and clinical associate Professor of Plastic Surgery).

Omnigraphics - Health Reference Series
Each volume in the Health Reference Series is written in concise, straightforward, Cosmetic and Reconstructive Surgery Sourcebook, 2nd edition ...
www.omnigraphics.com

Nicholas Perricone - Wikipedia, the free encyclopedia
Dr. Nicholas Perricone (pronounced /'pɛrɨkoʊn/), MD, is a dermatologist who has written several books, primarily on the subjects of weight loss
en.wikipedia.org/wiki/ Nicholas_Perricone

Arthur W. Perry, MD, FACS Plastic Surgery
22 Jul 2010 ... Order Straight Talk about Cosmetic Surgery, named the best health book of 2007 by ... And "Looking in the Mirror with Dr. Arthur Perry"
www.perryplasticsurgery.com

Chapter 2

Face and neck anatomy

Orbicularis oculi muscle

Orbicularis oculi muscle - Wikipedia, the free encyclopedia
The orbicularis oculi is a muscle in the face that closes the eyelids. The muscle acts to close the eye and is the only muscle capable of doing so. ...
en.wikipedia.org/wiki

Orbicularis Oculi Muscle of the Face and Eyes
Orbicularis oculi is a sphincter muscle around the eye and acts, in general, to narrow the eye opening and close the orbit of the eye. ...
www.face-and-emotion.com/dataface/expression/o_oculi.html

Oral Motor Assessment and Treatment 3810
Variety and control of movement for lips, cheeks, jaw, and tongue: Lowers the lower lips depressor anguli oris: lowers the bottom corner of the lips pterygoid (not shown): pulls jaw back or shut Mentalis: pulls chin down
www.slideshare.net

Oral Motor Assessment And Treatment 3810
Frontalis: the forehead corrugator: the brow Nasalis: the nose orbicularis oculi: around the eye levator labii: raises the upper lip masseter: closes the jaw ...
www.slideshare.net

Facial expression

The Lips
Rounding-spreading (the corners of the lips are drawn together or pulled apart). ...encircling the lips) and the Mentalis muscle (the muscle from the lower ... The depressor anguli oris muscles extend from the chin to the lower
www.linguistics.ucla.edu/people/ladefoge

Facial Muscles

The Facial Muscles
And in particular those in the lips help to shape the sound and air ...depressor anguli oris: lowers the bottom corner of the lips ... lips; pterygoid (not shown): pulls jaw back or shut; Mentalis: pulls chin down ...
www.yorku.ca/earmstro/journey/facial.html

Futurehealth
If such conduct does not make you soon feel cheerful, nothing else on that; Some zygomaticus muscles will be built up more around the front of their ... The eye muscles involved in smiling, the lower lateral orbicularis Oculi ... muscle of
www.futurehealth.org

The Magic Of Smiles And Laughter
These muscles are important to understand because the zygomatic majors are ... The orbicularis oculi at the eyes act independently and reveal the true feelings ... Lines around the eyes can also appear in intense fake smiles and the .... The Tight-Lipped Smile
westsidetoastmasters.com/resources

The mechanism of human facial expression
Tainted facial muscle tonus... One of the problems with Duchenne's theory is that it presumes the facial muscles to ...orbicularis oculi, was not said to be a smile of enjoyment...action of m. zygomaticus major was slight to moderate. .. and draws skin from around the eye inward (pars
www.paulekman.com

Paul Ekman - Emotions Revealed. Recognizing Faces and Feelings
Renowned expert in nonverbal communication Paul Ekman has led a renaissance in ...And I would work to develop an objective way to measure facial behavior so that any But sometimes our emotions get us into trouble.
www.scribd.com

Disorders of the voice - Telfort. ADSL internet provider
The voice, even without words, can express emotions such as the messages conveyed in an unintended way by body posture, movements, facial expression and voice have a ... The amount of non-verbal communication is grossly
home.tiscali.nl/knmg0234/VOICE.html

Nervous System
It automatically regulates heartbeat and controls muscle contractions in the walls... Facial, 7, Control most facial expressions; secretion of tears & saliva; the sense of taste and the sense of smell of each other; But if the alarming stimulus is repeated a
universe-review.ca/R10-16-ANS.htm

The Brain And Love
The Brain and Love Popular expressions reflect how we think about love. ..... Unlike telephone wires and poles, nerve cells do not touch each other; this emotional response allows us to move beyond our own survival and to help others. Subtle changes in facial
www.scribd.com

Facial expression - Wikipedia, the free encyclopedia
For instance, disgust and fear can be tough to tell apart; 3 Facial expressions; the muscles of facial expression; See also; References   External links. There are seven universally emotions shown through facial expressions: fear, anger,
en.wikipedia.org/wiki /Facial_expression

Confusions About Context in the Judgment of Facial Expression.
Judgment tasks, using clearly defined or well-understood emotional terms. The seven emotions shown of (anger, fear, disgust, contempt, surprise, sadness, happiness);
Disgust photo 1.Disgust photo 2. Disgust photo
www.paulekman.com/...content

Spanish basic emotion words are consistently ordered
Context, the detection of reliable phenomena in human constructions such as vocabularies is.... are clearly specified: 50% from Spain and 50% from America (of which, fear, sadness, surprise, happiness, anger, contempt and disgust
www.springerlink.com/index/m9306h75nm0083w5

ART NATOMY
The muscles of the head that act on the face are divided into two groups: those that move the skin of the face (the Subcutaneous Muscles) and those which move elements from the skeleton (the Masticators Muscles). ...They are distributed throughout the Region of the skull, the eyes, the nose,
www.artnatomia.net/uk/ARTNATOMYen.swf

A critical review of the literature of functional
These muscles are all intimately connected and no move- . These numbers can perhaps be divided into groups (Cooper In most muscles, the spindles are distributed through. The skin and ectodermal mucous membrane of the head,
ses.library.usyd.edu.au/bitstream/2123/4861/1/0029.pdf

Chapter 9 MuscularSystem
By contrast, the superficial fascia under the skin of the back of the hand, elbow, Flattened, sheet like tendons are called aponeurosis (ap"o˘ noo-ro'sez). Of Facial Expression* Muscle Epicranius Frontalis
www.scribd.com/doc/8752654/Chapter9MuscularSystem

Bones and Muscles
The galea aponeurotica travels over the top of the skull. And a side view of the skull showing the occipital bone and the mastoid process. .You saw a tiny aponeurosis in the eye lid. This one is a broad sheet that arises. They all converge into one tendon
www.scribd.com/doc/7204557/Bones-and-Muscles

Dr. Ben Bramwell
In other places, the tendons become long and flattened into a sheet like. Each of the muscle fibres attaching to the tendon attach at the same angle. ... Frontalis, Galea aponeurotica, Skin of the Eyebrow, Wrinkles forehead ... Occipitalis, Occipital
departments.weber.edu/zoology/Lecture9.htm

Flashcards Table on Human Anatomy Exam #2 Notes
Occipitalis muscle: name the Origin, Insertion and Action, O: occipital bone I: on galea aponeurotica A: orbicularis oculi muscle ... (medial 1/3) I: mastoid process A: bilateral: head to chest & unilateral: head rotation.... Femoris tendon;
www.proprofs.com/flashcards/tableview.php?title=human

Paul Ekman - Emotions Revealed. Recognizing Faces and Feelings
Renowned expert in nonverbal communication Paul Ekman has led a renaissance in. And I would work to develop an objective way to measure facial behavior so that any But sometimes our get us into trouble. That happens when our .It will also help
www.scribd.com

Disorders of the voice - Telfort. ADSL internet provider
The voice, even without words, can express emotions such as grief. The messages conveyed in an unintended way by body posture, movements, facial expression and voice have a ... The amount of non-verbal communication is grossly
home.tiscali.nl/knmg0234/VOICE.html

The Accessory Organs of the Eye - Gray's Anatomy of the Human
The movement of circumduction, as in looking around a room, is performed. The lateral angles are attached to the zygomatic bone by the lateral palpebral raphé. The orbital septum (septum
education.yahoo.com

Eyelid Anatomy: eMedicine Clinical Procedures
23 Nov 2009 ... Overview: The eyelids act to protect the anterior surface of the globe from local injury. Additionally, they aid in regulation of light reaching the eye, the orbital portion extends in a wide circular fashion around the
emedicine.medscape.com

Anatomy of the Eye (Ophthobook.com)
19 Dec 2007...The eyelids protect and help lubricate the eyes. The capsule is held in place by suspensory ligaments called zonules that insert around the periphery ... of the frontal bone, the zygomatic bone forms the strong lateral
www.ophthobook.com/chapters/anatomy

StateMaster - Encyclopedia: Muscle
Exercise has several effects upon muscles, connective tissue, bone; the external muscles of the eye are conspicuously large and strong in relation to. From fascia over the lower of the nasal bone Insertion/Distal Attachment: Part of the
www.statemaster.com/encyclopedia/Muscle

Physiology of adult Homo sapiens - Musculoskeletal apparatus and
Nasal bones (2) form the bridge of the nose and articulate with the...Composed of loose connective tissue and having a free smooth surface that lines .Procerus / Procerus muscle: origin, fascia over nasal bone; insertion, skin of forehead; innervations, facial; action, draws medial angle of eyebrows
www6.ufrgs.br/favet/imunovet/molecular.../muscles.

The A to Z of Skeletal *Muscles*
Collateral CSF = Cerebrospinal fluid CT = *connective tissue* e.g. = example EC ... Elion top of Epiphysis the end of a *long bone* beyond the growth plate (epiphyseal ... to the *eyebrow* pertaining to the outer wall of a cavity from paries,
www.scribd.com

Anatomy and Functions of the Muscles of Facial Expression
Its primary action is to draw down the medial angle of the eyebrows, This supraorbital bundle passes deep to the corrugator and turns upward across the ... The muscle fibers pass upward and laterally through the fibers of (A) Vertical glabelar wrinkling from
linkinghub.elsevier.com

Facial cutaneous reconstructive surgery: Facial flaps*** - Elsevier
After passing through the corrugator supercilii muscle, they lie in the deep ... This neurovascular bundle passes through the fibers of the frontalis muscle, Bone, and skin, is crucial for maintenance of its respiratory function. ... A series of furrows and wrinkle
linkinghub.elsevier.com

Eyebrow Ptosis
Medial margin of the frontalis. Its origin is from ... end of the eyebrow and produces horizontal wrinkles of the skin at the ... and eyebrow. The frontal branch (referred to in this figure and ... medial to the supraorbital bundle. .procerus-corrugator muscle complex
informahealthcare.com/doi/pdf/10.3109/08820539609063807

Informa Healthcare - Orbit
The frontalis muscle inserts into the brow skin after penetrating through the ... The corrugator supercilii muscle arises from the medial end of the orbit and runs ... All of these muscles depress the medial head of the eyebrow. Some patients will have over
informahealthcare.com

Paraoral Tissues
The border between the lips and the surrounding skin is referred to as the ... sphincters of the oral orifice o Buccinator o orbicularis oris anchor point for ... FUNCTIONS OF THE LIP Food intake Because they have their own muscles and ... Four paired intrinsic
www.scribd.com

Infraorbital nerve - definition of infraorbital nerve in the
Information about infraorbital nerve in free online English dictionary. Nerve into the eye socket, traversing the infraorbital canal to supply the upper incisors, .upper gums, lower eyelid and conjunctiva, and part of
dictionary.thefreedictionary.com/infraorbital+nerve

Head and neuroanatomy - Google Books Result
Wrinkles the root of the nose Narrows the naris (c) Elevates the upper lip and ... Orbicularis oris Buccinator Zygomaticus major Zygomaticus minor Risorius ...
books.google.co.uk

Anatomical basis for a safe and easier approach to composite...
Circumference by a plexus of small facial nerve branches. . Zygomaticus minor muscle and levator complex can be ... zygomaticus muscle (b) embedded by the SMAS layer. (c).deeply to the zygomaticus major muscle (a) and the thick... This fat lacks large
ww.springerlink.com

Variations in the facial muscles at the angle of the mouth
1, zygomaticus major m.; 2, zygomaticus minor m.; 3, in a large majority of the sides (83.5%) combining both of the races studied, (types B and C in Table 1). T h e converging point was found to be located either ... of the mouth only in a small
www3.interscience.wiley.com

Mastery of surgery - Google Books Result
Josef E. Fischer, K. I. Bland - 2007 - Medical ... b) levator anguli oris; c) zygomaticus major and minor; d) risorius; ... A small oral aperture also must be avoided because it
books.google.co.uk

Full text of "A dictionary of terms used in medicine and the ...
The employment ol the letter C, instead of the letter E, in terms of Greek ...... as depressor alas nasi, or my form is, muscle; depressor anguli oris,
www.archive.org/stream/.../adictionaryterm01hoblgoog

Full text of "The Century dictionary: an encyclopedic lexicon of ...
Capable ol Deing aetormea, capaoie 01 wei, e ^ COMeq uenta of...... Depressor anguli oris, or triangularis menti, a muscle of the face which draws down ...
www.archive.org/stream

Ptosis of the chin and lip incompetence: Consequences of lost...
The Mentalis muscle controls the posture of the chin. ... Its strength is altered only minimally by changes in chin position and is generally not a great surgical.... her primary concern related to distortion of the
linkinghub.elsevier.com/retrieve/pii/0278239189903376

The Mentalis muscle in relation to edentulous mandibles*1 - Elsevier
The Mentalis muscle acts to elevate the skin of the chin and causes the lower lip to ...Group A. In Group A, the lower lip of the cadaver was pulled
linkinghub.elsevier.com/retrieve/pii/0022391372902594

Explore Plastic Surgery - Dr. Barry Eppley
20 Oct 2009 ... The Effects of Chin Augmentation on Mentalis Muscle Strain and Lower LipIn competency ... Mentalis strain, as a result of the lips trying to come together, adding an implant is the only acceptable method of chin ...
exploreplasticsurgery.com/tag/mentalis-muscle-strain/

Alveolar process of maxilla: Facts, Discussion Forum,
In humans, the tooth-bearing bones are the maxilla. Maxilla ... The Buccinator is a thin quadrilateral muscle, occupying the interval between the maxilla and ... which aids in holding the cheek to the teeth during chewing.-Origin and. ...
www.absoluteastronomy.com

Anatomy - Scalp + face
Skin is thick, hair bearing and contains numerous sebaceous glands. ... These 14 bones form the basic shape of the face, and are responsible for providing ... Buccinator Upper fibers. Origin- from maxilla opposite molar teeth ...
www.slideshare.net/ananthatiger/anatomy-scalp-face

Spread of infection in facial space
5 Dec 2009... IF CONFINED TO BUCCINATOR: INFECTION DRAINS INTRA ORALLY IN BUCCAL VESTIBULE CROSSES Most jaw fractures in the tooth bearing segments are by ... OF LOOSE ALVEOLAR TISSUE
 www.docstoc.com/docs/.../spread-of-infection-in-fascial-space

Temporal muscle - Wikipedia, the free encyclopedia
The Temporalis; the zygomatic arch and Masseter have been removed. Latin, musculus temporalis. Origin temporal lines on the parietal bone of the skull. ...
en.wikipedia.org/wiki/Temporal muscle

Temporalis Muscle
An interactive animated tutorial on the muscle, including its attachments, actions,
www.getbodysmart.com

Temporal muscle: Information from Answers.com
Note: click on a word meaning below to see its connections and related words. The noun temporalis muscle has one meaning: Meaning #1: muscle.
www.answers.com/topic/temporalis-muscle

Medial pterygoid muscle - Wikipedia, the free encyclopedia
The Pterygoidei; the zygomatic arch and a portion of the ramus of the mandible ... The bulk of the muscle arises as a deep head from just above the medial ... Like the lateral pterygoid, and all other muscles of mastication (apart from
en.wikipedia.org/wiki/Medial_pterygoid_muscle

Functional anatomy of the human lateral pterygoid muscle
Short and squat, the lateral pterygoid muscle (pterygoideus lateralis) has the general form.... view showing the deep variation of the maxillary artery. ...
www.springerlink.com/index/p6m62k7173570612.pdf

The Head - Human Anatomy
In anatomy, the head of an animal is the rostral part (from anatomical position) ... The upper border of the ramus of mandible is thin, and is surmounted by two ... of the head) that cover the inferior and medial to the eye socket (or orbit)
www.slideshare.net/examville/997610-anatomyhead - United States

Head and neck anatomy - Wikipedia, the free encyclopedia
Move head, Splenius capitis, dorsal rami of middle and lower cervical nerves ... Blood circulates from the upper systemic loop originating at the aortic arch, Knowledge of anatomy of nerves and other vital structures in the head and .. Anterior: fossae (Incisive
en.wikipedia.org/wiki/Head_and_neck_anatomy

Anatomy Tables - Parotid Gland & Face
inf. labial as., lat. nasal br., angular a. lower part of palatine tonsil, ... septal br. lower nasal septum; upper lip - skin, muscles & mucosa ... skin of the face, anastomoses with branches of the buccal, infraorbital and facial arteries ... in superficial
anatomy.med.umich.edu/nervous_system/face_tables.html

Full text of "The Century dictionary: an encyclopedic lexicon of ...
Depressor labii inferioris, or qitadratus menti, a muscle of the face which draws down the lower lip. Depressor mandibulas, the depressor of the mandible,
www.archive.org/stream/.../centurydictipt600whituoft_djvu.txt

Platysma muscle - Wikipedia, the free encyclopedia
The platysma is a superficial muscle that overlaps the sternocleidomastoid. It is a broad sheet arising from the fascia covering the upper parts of the
en.wikipedia.org/wiki/Platysma_muscle

What is the Platysma Muscle?
12 Sep 2008 ... The Platysma Muscle is a facial muscle. It is a broad sheet of muscle arising... When all the fibers of the platysma muscle work together,
www.squidoo.com/platysma_muscle

What is the Platysma Muscle?
Have you ever heard of the Platysma muscle? If not then you would not be alone! However, if you suffer from a double chin then you may
hubpages.com/hub/What-is-the-Platysma-Muscle

Sternocleidomastoid muscle - Wikipedia, the free encyclopedia
The triangles of the neck. (Anterior triangles to the left; posterior triangles to the right.) Sternocleidomastoideus.png. Muscles of the
en.wikipedia.org/wiki/Sternocleidomastoid_muscle

File:Sternocleidomastoideus.png - Wikipedia, the free encyclopedia
File:Sternocleidomastoideus.png. From Wikipedia, the free encyclopedia. Jump to: navigation, search. File; File history; File links;
en.wikipedia.org/wiki/File%3ASternocleidomastoideus.png

Musculus sternocleidomastoideus - definition of musculus...
Noun, musculus sternocleidomastoideus - one of two thick muscles running from the sternum and clavicle to the mastoid and occipital
www.thefreedictionary.com/musculus

Did you know you have more than 600 muscles in your body?
They do everything from pumping blood throughout your body to helping you lift your heavy
kidshealth.org › How the Body Works

Muscle building - most effective weightlifting routines, exercises...
The most effective muscle building exercises are compound movements. Compound movements are exercises that require your body to use more than one muscle. ...
www.intense-workout.com/muscle_building.html

Free Muscle Building Presentation
In addition to everything else, you'll also receive free lifetime updates on "The Muscle Gain Truth No-Fail System." As I add even more
www.musclegaintruth.comsternocleidomastoideus

Human Physiology - Muscle
Muscle cells, ensheathed by endomysium, consist of many fibrils (or ... Skeletal muscles may be made up of hundreds or even thousands, of muscle fibers ... Each bundle of muscle fiber is called a fasciculus and is surrounded by a layer ... on the sarcolemma
people.eku.edu/ritchisong/301notes3.htm

Zebrafish periostin is required for the adhesion of muscle fiber...
Muscle fibers do not attach to bones and cartilages directly, and in the attachment ... Thin layers of tissue, connective endomysium, perimysium, and epimysium (fascia), which lap each muscle fiber, a group of muscle fibers, and
linkinghub.elsevier.com/retrieve/pii/S0012160603007875

Directional terms describe the positions of human structures...
13 Sep 2006 .The tendons of *many muscles* extend over joints and in this way .*Each bundle* of *muscle fiber* is called a *fasciculus* and is *surrounded* by a layer of connective tissue called the *perimysium* ... Tendon: Commonly, the epimysium, *perimysium*,
web.njit.edu/.../IE665/Muscle%20and%20nerve%20-1%20small.doc

Microsoft PowerPoint - chap 9-*muscle tissue*
Packed by *connective tissue* sheets into *skeletal muscles* –
Hundreds to *thousands* in a *single muscle fiber*. • *make up* 80% of *cell* volume ...
www.montgomerycollege.edu/.../chap%209_muscle%20tissue

Skeletal Muscle
Fascia, connective tissue outside the epimysium, surrounds and separates the muscles. Portions of the epimysium project inward to divide the muscle into compartments. Each compartment contains a bundle of muscle fibers.
www.afitrainer.com/become-a-personal-trainer.

Human Physiology - Muscle
Fascia, connective tissue outside the epimysium, surrounds and separates the muscles. Portions of the epimysium project inward to divide the muscle into compartments. Each compartment contains a bundle of muscle fibers. Each bundle of muscle fiber is called a fasciculus and is surrounded by a
people.eku.edu/ritchisong/301notes3.htm

Lecture III
Fascia, connective tissue outside the epimysium, surrounds and separates the muscles. Portions of the epimysium project inward to divide the muscle into compartments. ... Each compartment contains a bundle of muscle fibers. Each bundle of muscle fiber is called a fasciculus and is
faculty.ksu.edu.sa/68417/Documents/Lecture%20III%20relaxation.ppt

Directional terms describe the positions of human structures...
Fascia, connective tissue outside the epimysium, surrounds and separates the muscles. Portions of the epimysium project inward to divide the muscle into compartments. Each compartment contains a bundle of muscle fibers. Each bundle of muscle fiber is called a
web.njit.edu/.../IE665/Muscle%20and%20nerve%20-1%20smal

The Concise Book of Muscles Chris Jarmey - 2008
The place where a muscle attaches to a relatively stationary point on a bone, either directly or via a tendon is called the origin. When the
books.google.co.uk/books?isbn=1556437196

Skeletal Muscle and Fascia
7 Jan 2010The place where a muscle attaches to a relatively stationary point on a bone, either directly or via a tendon is called the origin. ...
www.docstoc.com/docs/21554231/Skeletal-Muscle-and-Fascia

Chapter 10 An Analysis of Bone/Muscle Movement
Bone is composed of structural units called Haversian systems. (a) Origin: attached by tendons to a stationary bone. (b) Insertion: attached .Attach the spring scales to positions 2 and 3 and adjust
www.ableweb.org/volumes/vol-15/10-jacklet

Spatial heterogeneity in the muscle functional
MRI signal this was proposed to affect the pH change through a relatively greater; given the demonstrated importance of muscle fiber type to the T2 change of ... we were not able to find data in the literature to either support or refute .Non uniform strain of
linkinghub.elsevier.com/retrieve/pii/S0730725X08000519

Connective tissue morphogenesis by fibroblast traction by D Stopak
Based on our comparisons of the forces exerted by various cell types during ... Dense bundles of aligned collagen fibers form tendons connecting muscles to which have been aligned circumferentially and wrap around the explant. The cells themselves
linkinghub.elsevier.com/retrieve/pii/0012160682903888

All about Health and Body - CSS Forums
The body is made up of three types of muscle tissue: skeletal. Every day, the average person's muscles work as hard as if they were placing 2400 pounds on a .This tapers to a tendon that rounds the elbow and attaches to. Cells are bent by
www.cssforum.com.pk/...notes/11811-all-about-health-body.html

20A Lecture notes - Chapter One The Human Body: An Orientation
Tissue Types. Epithelial
Tissue. II. Connective.
Tissue 2. Neuromuscular junction
elaney.org/wp/amy_bohorquez

BIOMEDICAL ENGINEERING AND DESIGN HANDBOOK, Fundamentals
Incident light is carried to the *tissue* by *fiber* optic cables, where it is scattered by the ......*muscle* is called the *neuromuscular junction*. One
www.4electron.com/ftp/hons/biomedhan/01.pdf

Rehabilitation of Sports Injuries - Scientific Basis
Begird and e. fink *4 Tissue* Healing and Repair: *Tendons* and Ligaments, *Details* of the *muscle* show: (A) a degenerative
Myofibril - Wikipedia, the free encyclopedia

Myofibril - Definition
The muscle cell is nearly filled with myofibrils running parallel to each other on the long axis of the cell. The sarcomeric subunits of one
www.wordiq.com/definition/Myofibril

Myosin - Wikipedia, the free encyclopedia
This protein makes up part of the sarcomere and forms macromolecular filaments Similar filament-forming myosin proteins were found in cardiac muscle, ... the side of the thick filament, ready to walk along the adjacent actin-based thin ... Myosin VI is an
en.wikipedia.org/wiki/Myosin

Actin, Myosin, and Cell Movement -- The Cell -- NCBI Bookshelf
Myosin is the prototype of a molecular motor—a protein that converts (B) Diagram showing the organization of actin (thin) and myosin (thick) filaments in the thick filaments of muscle consist of several hundred myosins. In non-muscle cells and in
www.ncbi.nlm.nih.gov

Myosins Move Along Actin Filaments -- Biochemistry -- NCBI...
Muscle contraction depends on the motion of thin filaments (blue).The thick filaments have diameters of about 15 nm (150 Å) and consist primarily of myosin. For example, actin sequestering proteins such as thymosin bind to actin ... showing that individual
www.ncbi.nlm.nih.gov

Nerve Cell (Neuronal) Synapse with Muscle Fiber (Neuromuscular ...
Nerve Cell (Neuronal) Synapse with Muscle Fiber (Neuromuscular Junction) - Medical ...Nucleus Medical Media creates and/or licenses medical illustrations
catalog.nucleusinc.co

Muscle - Wikipedia, the free encyclopedia
There are two broad types of voluntary muscle fibers: slow twitch and fast twitch. .... Muscle is mainly composed of muscle cells. Within the cells are myofibrils ... movement by direct connections with the efferent nerves in the spine
en.wikipedia.org/wiki/Muscle

Acetylcholine receptor - Wikipedia, the free encyclopedia
An acetylcholine receptor (abbreviated AChR) is an integral membrane protein that responds to the binding of acetylcholine, a neurotransmitter. ...
en.wikipedia.org/wiki/Acetylcholine receptor

Control of acetylcholine receptors in skeletal muscle
May be enhanced by the fixed localization in the membrane. . The nicotinic acetylcholine receptor (AChR) is a pentameric glycol protein Reconstitution experiment incorporating the
www.springerlink.com/index/R72682102H642665.

What is a Cell
Organelles are found only in eukaryotes and are always surrounded by a protective membrane. ... It houses the cell's chromosomes and is the place where almost all... how food and nutrients are turned into energy packets and water.
www.ncbi.nlm.nih.gov/About/primer/genetics_cell.html

Hot Video: mitochondria
Mitochondria are the cell's power producers. They convert energy into forms that are ...Mitochondria: Normal structures responsible for energy production in cells. ... Inside our cells – powerhouses that use oxygen to generate power is a membrane-enclosed
www.williambrosbrew.com/catalog

Cell: Definition from Answers.com
A single unit that converts radiant energy into electric energy: a solar cell... One of the most prominent organelles within a eukaryotic cell is the nucleus. The endoplasmic reticulum is composed of membrane-enclosed flattened sacs. The power-houses of the,
www.answers.com/topic/cell

Muscle contraction - Wikipedia, the free encyclopedia
While nerve impulse profiles are, for the most part, always the same: Exercise that incorporates both eccentric and concentric muscular contractions ... can produce greater gains in strength than
en.wikipedia.org/wiki/Muscle contraction

Muscle Hypertrophy - Definition
When someone starts exercising a muscle there is first an increase in the nerve impulses that cause muscle contraction. This alone often results in strength gains without any noticeable change in muscle size. As one continues to exercise, there is a complex
sportsmedicine.about.com/od/glossar

Muscle contraction: Definition from Answers.com
Muscle contraction the electrochemical process of generating tension within a muscle. ..The muscle changes length and takes a joint through a specific range of; While nerve impulse profiles are, for the
www.answers.com/topic/muscle-contraction

Cellular respiration - Wikipedia, the free encyclopedia
Aerobic respiration requires oxygen in order to generate energy (ATP).The chemical process store less energy than the reactants and the reaction ...The yields in the table below are for one glucose molecule being fully oxidized into carbon
en.wikipedia.org/wiki/Cellular respiration

Metabolism - Wikipedia, the free encyclopedia
The chemical reactions of metabolism are organized into metabolic ... Enzymes are crucial to metabolism because they allow organisms to drive desirable reactions that require: This oxidation releases carbon dioxide as a waste product. .
en.wikipedia.org/wiki/Metabolism

Global Health & Fitness - Exercise
Your muscles take in a source of energy and they use it to generate force. ... T hey need oxygen, because chemical reactions require ATP and oxygen is consumed to produce ATP. They need to eliminate metabolic wastes (carbon dioxide, lactic acid) As ATP gets
www.globalhealthandfitness.com/exercise.htm

How Stuff Works "How Exercise Works"
Your muscles take in a source of energy and *they* use it to *generate* ... They need oxygen, because chemical reactions require ATP and oxygen is consumed to produce ATP. They need to eliminate metabolic wastes *(carbon dioxide, lactic acid)* ... As the work of the muscle increases, more and more ATP gets *consumed* and ...
www.howstuffworks.com

Cell Volume and Muscle Growth
The larger the cells, the larger the overall muscle, it's that simple. Muscle fiber hyperplasia + Muscle fiber hypertroph *many* big muscle fibers. The *overall size* of the balloon *larger (increase* in contractile protein).This enables the *muscle* glutamine to
www.ironmagazine.com/article581.html

Muscle Fiber Hypertrophy *vs.* Hyperplasia
Hypertrophy refers to an increase in the *size* of the *cell* while *hyperplasia refers to:* controls despite the fact that the *overall size* of the deltoid *muscle* was greater. ... These new myoblastic *cells* can either fuse with an existing *muscle fiber* causing that fiber to get
www.realx3mforum.com/smf/index.php?topic=17367.0

Muscle - Wikipedia, the free encyclopedia
During development, myoblasts (*muscle* progenitor *cells*) either *remain* in the somite to ... fibers are pulling at an angle to the *overall* action of the *muscle*, be *increased* through exercise; instead the *muscle cells simply* get *bigger*. *Muscle fibers* have a limited capacity
en.wikipedia.org/wiki/Muscle

Training for *Size* and Strength: Advanced Training Planning for...
Most recently we discussed the role of satellite *cells* in *muscle* growth of quality research looking specifically at *muscle hypertrophy* in humans using typical ... *Muscle* strength, *fiber size*, and surface EMG activity of the quadriceps
www.thinkmuscle.com/articles/haycock/training-03.htm

Muscle contraction: Definition from Answers.com
Classification of voluntary muscular contractions. Skeletal muscle contractions can be broadly separated into twitch and tetanic contractions. ...
www.answers.com/topic/muscle-contraction

Muscle contraction - Wikipedia, the free encyclopedia
1 Contractions, by muscle type. 1.1 Skeletal muscle contractions. 1.1.1 Classification of voluntary muscular contractions. 1.2 Smooth muscle contraction ...
en.wikipedia.org/wiki/Muscle contraction

Isometric exercise

Isometric Exercises for Static Strength Training
Isometric exercises can be used for general strength conditioning and for rehabilitation. Also known as static strength training, involve muscular actions ...
www.sport-fitness-advisor.com/isometric-exercises

Isometric Exercises. Its Advantages and Disadvantages.
Incorporated isometric exercises in your everyday life and in your regular flat belly workout and get all the benefits of isometric movements.
www.flat-belly-exercises.com/isometric-exercises.html

Bodybuilding.com - The Charles Atlas Workout Revisited! - Kelly...
This is an example of an isometric movement. It turns out Isometric exercises have several benefits for both strength athletes and bodybuilders. ...
www.bodybuilding.com

Isotonic exercises

Isotonic (exercise physiology) - Wikipedia, the free encyclopedia
In an isotonic contraction, tension remains unchanged and the muscle's length changes. Lifting an object at a constant speed is an example of isotonic...
en.wikipedia.org/.../Isotonic (exercise physiology)

Different exercise types of contraction isometric, concentric...
All lifting exercises require isotonic contractions. This happens when the muscle shortens as it contracts. An example of isotonic contraction can be seen ...
www.weightlossforall.com/exercise-types

A weight-lifting exercise model for inducing hypertrophy in the...
A weight-lifting exercise model for inducing hypertrophy in the hind limb ... of isotonic high-intensity, short-duration, and graded overload exercises. ...
www.ncbi.nlm.nih.gov/pubmed/1406173

Build your Body Free Health Fitness Tips Exercise
It can take as long as two months for actual hypertrophy to begin. The additional contractile proteins ... All lifting exercises are isotonic contractions. ...
changeyourlooks.net/bldyourbdy/buildbody

Geriatric rehabilitation manual
Timothy L. Kauffman, John O. Barr, Michael L. Moran - 2007 - Health & Fitness - 559 pages
The benefits of strength training with isometric, isotonic and isokinetic routines
have ...Hypertrophy occurs even in individuals aged 90 years and above, ...
books.google.co.uk/books?isbn=0443102333...

Muscle - Wikipedia, the free encyclopedia
The exact cause of sarcopenia is unknown, but it may be due to a combination of the
gradual ... cells" which help to regenerate skeletal muscle fibers, and a decrease in sensitivity to or
the availability of critical secreted growth factors which are necessary to
en.wikipedia.org/wiki/

Muscle atrophy
The branched-chain amino acids or BCAAs *(leucine,* isoleucine, and valine) are critical to this
process, in addition to lysine and other amino acids. ...
www.philippines-bohol.info/Muscle atrophy

DBExtraction - Health and Fitness, bodybuilding supplements, diet...
60% of free-form *amino acids* floating in *skeletal muscles* is L-glutamine. .. As well as 5 grams
of *BCAAs* (*leucine, isoleucine, and valine*) in each scoop! ...
www.healthnutwarehouse.com/extraction.html

The modulation of caveolin-1 expression controls *satellite cell*
Satellite cell activation during *muscle repair.* Dani Volonte,* Youhua Liu,† and ...membranes,
contributes to signaling *events* that lead to activation of *satellite cells* during ....conclude that
activation of the signaling *cascade* ... caveolin-1 *activates*
www.fasebj.org/cgi/reprint/19/2/237.pdf

Satellite cell-mediated angiogenesis in vitro coincide
by RP Rhoads – 2009 Leading to fibrosis in the muscle core due to the loss of myogenic cells Such
evidence indicates that muscle repair requires that myogenesis and ... Normally quiescent in adult
skeletal muscle, satellite cells activate upon muscle. Under normal conditions, a cascade of
www.ncbi.nlm.nih.gov/pmc/articles/PMC2692418/

High concentrations of HGF inhibit skeletal muscle satellite cell
By M Yamada – 2010 The subsequent signal transduction cascade of common intracellular...The
role of HGF in muscle repair, however, may not be restricted to: Hepatocyte growth factor
activates quiescent skeletal muscle satellite cells in vitro.
ajpcell.physiology.org/cgi/content/full/298/3/C465

International review of cell and molecular biology arab2000
Introduction Caveolae are specialized sub domains of the plasma membrane found in most
cell types, and particularly abundant in highly differentiated cells.
www.scribd.com/.../international-review-of-cell-and-molecular-biology

Chapter 3

Facial toning Exercises

Sarcopenia

Sarcopenia - Wikipedia, the free encyclopedia
Sarcopenia (from the Greek meaning "poverty of flesh") is the degenerative loss of skeletal muscle
mass and strength associated
en.wikipedia.org/wiki/Sarcopenia

Sarcopenia
Sarcopenia can be defined as the age-related loss of muscle mass, strength and function (Waters, Baumgartner & Garry 2000; Vandervoort & Symons 2001). .
www.unm.edu/~lkravitz/Article%20folder/sarcopenia.html

Sarcopenia ~ Where strength equals freedom
Jun 23, 2010 At *sarcopenia*.com I seek to report on any issues that further our knowledge of *sarcopenia* and obesity
www.sarcopenia.com

What Are You Doing to Fight *Sarcopenia*? – Health Steps Rx
May 6, 2008 ... Just like osteoporosis and arthritis, "*sarcopenia* is a serious degenerative condition that increases ones risks for falls and
www.healthstepsrx.com/resources/articles/sarcopenia.htm

How Stuff Works "What's *sarcopenia* and what can you do about it?"
Apr 23, 2009 ... *Sarcopenia* is the loss of muscle mass and coordination that results from the process of aging. See the causes of *sarcopenia* and how it can
health.howstuffworks.com

Internal abuse

Long-term effects of *alcohol* - Wikipedia, the free encyclopedia
This effect is *not* unique to *alcohol but* can *also* occur with long term use of drugs which have a similar mechanism of action to *alcohol such* as the.... Chronic excessive *alcohol*
en.wikipedia.org/wiki/Long-term_effects_of_alcohol

Aging, Drugs, and *Alcohol*: Encyclopedia of Drugs, *Alcohol*, and...
In Western society, *smoking* cigarettes and excessive drinking of *alcohol* are two of the ...*Alcohol* and drug *abuse causes* thousands of *premature* deaths, *Alcohol not only* produces inflammation of the stomach *but also* increases the ... while taking
www.enotes.com/drugs-alcoho

External abuse

Sunburn - Wikipedia, the free encyclopedia
Sunburn is a burn to living tissue, such as skin, which is produced by overexposure to ultraviolet (UV) radiation, commonly from the sun's
en.wikipedia.org/wiki/Sunburn

Sunburn Causes, Symptoms, Diagnosis, and Treatment on...
Sunburn results from too much sun or sun-equivalent exposure. ... Although seldom fatal (sun poisoning), *sunburn* can be disabling and cause quite a bit of ...
www.emedicinehealth.com

Sunburn - Introduction
Information on *Sunburn* from NHS. Choices including causes, symptoms, diagnosis, risks and treatment and with links to other useful resources.
www.nhs.uk/conditions/sunburn

P&G Beauty & Grooming | The Dermis
Beneath the epidermis lies a much thicker *skin layer*, the *dermis*. ... Both *collagen* and elastin fibers are made by *cells* called *fibroblasts, as we get* older the amount of hyaluronic acid produced in the
www.pgbeautygroomingscience.com

Gen III skin care. Beyond mere "moisturizing" and sun protection...
In the *dermis*, the *lower* structural *layer* of the *skin*, lies one of the ... *Fibroblasts* in the *dermis* create *collagen* fibers and control the makeup and ... *As we age*, *cell* turnover in the
www.natural-health-information-centre.com/gen-iii-skin-care.html -

Treating Wrinkles - Anti Aging Shield
Photo damage is harmful to the *skin because* it releases collagenase enzymes. *Dermis* - Bottom *layer of skin* - Much thicker – Approximately 1000 microns (10 x ... Thick *layer* of structural tissue, primarily *collagen* (made by *Fibroblast cells*) .... During *skin's* regular
www.bioskinregeneration.com/wrinkles

NaturalRussia.com: Skin structure: Natural Russia
A *skin cell* starts its life at the *lower layer* of the *skin* (the basal *layer* of the ... This process speeds up *as we age*. *Dermis*. The *dermis* is the *layer* ... never reach the *dermis because collagen* and elastin molecules are too large ... The proper function
www.naturalrussia.com/natural/skin/structure

All About Skin
As these *cells get* closer to the *skin's* surface, they become larger, the stratum corneum is also referred to as the "horny *layer*," *because* its *cells* ... new *cells* are put in place, but this shedding process slows down *as we age*. ... That holds
www.skincare-answers.com/skin.html

Sagging Skin and Loose Facial Muscles - Skin Help (UK)
To add to the problem, the *muscles* in our face are *also* weakened by *age* so ... Sun exposure, smoking, and weight *loss* all contribute to the development of ...
www.skinhelp.co.uk/SaggingSkinAndLooseFacialMuscles.html

The *Aging* Face - NH, New Hampshire, *MA, Massachusetts*
Clues to *Facial Aging* Major forces responsible for *facial aging* include sun damage ... and the *muscles* underneath the fat weaken and lose elasticity and tone. ... Surgery after massive weight *loss* and tummy tucks. We *also* offer *facial* ...
www.plasticsurgerypa.com/index.cfm?event

Slackened facial tendons

Face Lift - Hillstrom Facial Plastic Surgery - Robert P. Hillstrom...
The muscles on the neck can *slacken*, too, causing you to look years older ... of the face called the SMAS, and it's *ligamentous* attachments are released, ...
www.hillstromplasticsurgery.com/pro_facelift.php

Collagen fibre orientation in the annulus fibrosus of...
Facet joints, longitudinal *ligaments* and extra- neous flesh were removed. .... tilt of the *slackened* fibers to decrease by 2.7 (assuming the dorsal-ventral ...
linkinghub.elsevier.com/retrieve/pii/0304416582903129

BOTOX, Facelift, Nose Job - *Facial* Surgery Procedures
The jaw line *slackens*, and folds and fat deposits appear on the neck. , of skin (the dermis) which "plumps up" the skin, joints, bones and *ligaments*. .... Chin surgery helps provide a harmonious balance to your *facial* features so ...
www.drandrewamunategui.com/aa-face.html

Facial Therapies - Anantara
This unique organ has 52 bones, 66 joints, 214 *ligaments*, 38 muscles and ... Elemis Oxygen Skin Calm *Facial* ... For aging, stressed and *slackened* skin. ...
spa.anantara.com/maldives/Facials/default.aspx

Slackened facial tendons

Brown's syndrome - Wikipedia, the free encyclopedia
Brown syndrome is caused by a malfunction of the superior oblique *tendon* sheath. ... Is described as the *tendon-slackening* from its center attachment to the.... *Facial* reconstruction is the final option to help patients with
en.wikipedia.org/wiki/Brown's syndrome

FAQ - Facefirm Facial Exercise Programme
Even really wasted muscle can work again so although your *facial* muscles are dormant you... (Unlike the rest of the body where the muscles attach to bone or *tendon*). ... To prevent the muscles at the side of your face from *slackening* and losing
www.facefirm.com/faq.php5

Meronk - Canthopexy and Lower Eyelid Surgery
Just as *facial* surgeons have begun to appreciate the superiority of volume restoration and preservation over ... The lid then undergoes a subtle realignment and *slackening*. Canthopexy strengthens and stabilizes the canthal tendon.
www.drmeronk.com

Thin skin

What Are the Causes of Thinning *Skin*? | eHow.com
There are some medical conditions that can cause the skin to thin, *according to* ...including Ehler's-Danlos syndrome, Frohlich syndrome, Cushing syndrome, Goltz syndrome, adrenal cancer, Cockayne Syndrome, Daentl-Townsend Syndrome,Fontaine-
www.ehow.com

Thin skin - WrongDiagnosis.com
The following *medical conditions* are *some* of the possible *causes* of *thin skin*. *There* are.... from Fibronectin Abnormality ... *thin skin*; *Ehlers-Danlos syndrome*, cardiac valvular form ... *thin skin* ... *thin skin*; *Growth Hormone Receptor* Deficiency
www.wrongdiagnosis.com/sym/thin_skin.htm

Very Thin *Skin*
Some ways to deal with very thin *skin*. ... Where the radio waves had penetrated to the subcutaneous *fat layer* and literally melted away facial *fat pads*. ...
www.ageless-beauty.com

Structure and Function: Biology of the *Skin*: Merck Manual Home
The *skin* has three *layers*—the epidermis, dermis, and *fat layer* (also called the subcutaneous *layer*). Each *layer* performs specific tasks. .
www.merck.com/mmhe/sec18/ch201/ch201b.html

Loss of facial bone

Facial bone loss contributes to aging
Facial bone loss contributes to *aging*. Study: CAT scans show shrinking volume to blame for wrinkled skin. You can blame the bones in the face,
www.online-ambulance.com/articles/grp/Senior/.../Fbonel.htm

Facial Bones Change With Age - Consumer Guide to Plastic Surgery
Learn how your *facial* bones change with *age* and what to do about sagging *facial* ... volume in areas of *bone loss*, such as *facial* fillers or injectables. ...
www.yourplasticsurgeryguide.com/facial.../facial-bones.htm

Study reveals facial bone changes add to aging appearance
24 Mar 2010 ... This *loss* of bony volume may contribute sagging facial skin, changes in *facial bone* structure as people *age* gives physicians new insight ...
www.news-medical.net

Strong Bones
Here's how the low-fat, high calcium *Strong Bones* Diet, when combined with an active lifestyle, can help make and keep your bones strong: • Dairy foods.
www.ivillage.com/

Foods for Strong Bones | Life Mojo
Foods for Strong Bones - If you think brittle bones are just for old people, you've got a lot to bone up on. True, osteoporosis usually affects women after ...
www.lifemojo.com

Eat these foods for strong bones TODAY Health
Don't let your bones get weak. Food Network dietitian Ellie Krieger has food dos and don'ts for protecting and taking care of your *bones*.
today.msnbc.msn.com/id/19613906/ - United States

Breakfasts for *Strong Bones*: 12 *Foods* to Boost Bone Health
Diagnosed with osteoporosis? Getting the calcium and vitamin D you need is easier than you think -- if you think better breakfasts!
www.webmd.com/osteoporosis/living-with.../diet-nutrition

Elastin & collagen fibers

Cutaneous disorders: Dermal disorders
Proteins with a long half-life, *collagen* and *elastin*, are subject to ... The dermo-epidermal junction is flatter since the papillae are *less* numerous. ... Roughness, *loose* skin, pigmentation, from the effects of UVA irradiation on ... *Elastin fibers* are normally
www.loreal.com/_en/_ww/.../desordres_dermiques.aspx

Skin Physiology and *Elastin*
Scar tissue is composed of *collagen fibers*. *Elastin* fibers [found in the ... Everyone, whether female or male, will begin to *lose* skin *elastin* fibers at age 25. confirm that our skin produces/synthesizes *less* and *less elastin* fibers ...
www.ethocyninfo.com/skinphysi.php

Blue Histology - Connective Tissues
8 Jun 2009 ... *Collagen* and *elastic fibers* intermingle in the dermis, i.e. the ... Fat cells or adipocytes are fixed cells in *loose* connective.... In brown adipose tissue, the nuclei of adipocytes are round and located more or *less* ...
www.lab.anhb.uwa.edu.

Collagen & Elastin Articles | Natural Skin Care
9 Jul 2010 ... Chronic inflammation degrades the *elastic collagen fibers*. ... The skin becomes *less* firm and *less elastic*. ... As the skin becomes *loose*, these creases that would normally be stretched out by the *elastic* fibers become
www.defendyour

How To Reverse Sun Damaged Skin
And advice on how to reverse the damage ... the greater its *healing* ability will be and the *slower* your skin will *age*. ...
www.eruptingmind.com/how-to-reverse-sun-damaged-skin/

Slower healing of damaged skin

Diagnose-Me: Condition: Poor/*Slow* Wound *Healing*
20 Jul 2010 ... Poor/*Slow* Wound *Healing* suggests the following may be present: ....Complications are more likely to develop in *aging skin*,
www.diagnose-me.com/cond/C233696.htm

New Hope For *Aging* And *Damaged Skin* Comes From Apple Stem
9 Feb 2010 ... New Hope for Aging and Damaged Skin Comes from Apple Stem Cells ...sophisticated measures such as stem cell *healing* and tissue reproduction. ... If a problem exists, it is the *slow* regeneration procedure the epidermal ...
www.immortalhumans.com

The Biology of *Skin, Aging* Damage, Sun Damage, the Epidermis
Aging and Sun *Damaged Skin* Development of Common Skin Lesions *Age* Spots.... and there is a *slower* turnover of the surface
www.skinbiology.com/skinhealth&aging.html

Uncommon organic activator of tissue *healing* & *skin* regeneration...
Evidence of *Aging*: Changes in Physiology *Skin aging* derives from the ... UV exposure can also penetrate the *skin*, damage basal cells, and *slow* down the speed.... *skin* is *damaged*, particularly in younger people, where *skin* injuries *heal* ...
www.bioskinregeneration.com/aging

Intrinsic ageing

Causes of Aging Skin
20 Jun 2005 ... Aging caused by the genes we inherit is called intrinsic (internal) aging. ...*Intrinsic aging*, also known as the natural aging process ...
www.skincarephysicians.com/agingskinnet/basicfacts.html

Intrinsic Aging - Anti-Aging Information – Anti aging skin care...
Anti -aging - *intrinsic aging* information including dry and thin skin, fine wrinkles, abnormal blood vessels, age spots, benign and malignant skin tumors.
www.anti-aging-guide.co.uk/skin-aging-symptoms.html

Intrinsic Aging - The Natural Aging Process
30 May 2008 ... Intrinsic aging, also known as the natural aging process, is a continuous process that normally begins in our mid-20s.
ezinearticles.com/? Intrinsic-Aging-

Intrinsic and Extrinsic Aging - Beauty Basics
There are two types of aging that you should be aware of. Intrinsic aging, you have no control over. Extrinsic aging is all about you and
www.bellaonline.com/articles/art32528.asp

Disease*: Definition, Synonyms from Answers.com
After that is the first extrinsic disease entry on the list, number 6, pneumonia and.....Subjective manifestations of a disease process such as weakness, pain ... Thus the definition, treatment, and
www.answers.com/topic/disease

Women love beauty » Blog Archive » Intrinsic Aging & Extrinsic
Extrinsic (external) aging is also intrinsic aging compounded by external ... caused by harsh detergents, rough treatment, cosmetics and disease processes. ...
womenlovebeauty.com/beauty-tips/anti-aging/5347

Aging skin how to a just your daily regimen
There are many *causes* for your skin to age. Some we have control over
others ...*Extrinsic* (*external*) aging is intrinsic aging compounded by *external causes* ... caused by harsh detergents, *rough treatment*, cosmetics, and disease
www.natural-skin-care-info.com/Aging-skin.html

Photoageing

Aging skin, cutaneous aging, *and photoageing*.
15 Jun 2009 ... Aging skin, cutaneous aging, *and photoaging*. Authoritative facts about the skin from the New Zealand Dermatological Society.
dermnetnz.org/site-age-specific/aging.html - New Zealand

Photoaging - Definition of Photoagaing - Aging Skin
27 Apr 2008 ... *Photoaging* refers to the damage that is done to the skin from prolonged exposure, over a person's lifetime, to UV
dermatology.about.com/od/glossary/g/photoaging.htm

Definition of matrix *metalloproteinase* - NCI Dictionary of Cancer...
Because these enzymes need zinc or calcium atoms to work properly, they are called *metalloproteinases*. Matrix *metalloproteinases* are involved in
www.cancer.gov/dictionary/?CdrID=44211

Matrix metalloproteinases*: a review.
Matrix *metalloproteinases* (MMPs) are a family of nine or more highly homologous Zn (++)-endopeptidases that collectively cleave most if not all of the ...
www.ncbi.nlm.nih.gov/pubmed/8435466

Matrix *Metalloproteinases* and Tissue Inhibitors of...
Matrix *metalloproteinases* (MMPs), also designated matrixins, hydrolyze components of the extracellular matrix. These proteins play a central role in many ...
circres.ahajournals.org/cgi/content/full/92/8/827

Inhibition of matrix *metalloproteinases*: a new *skin* care frontier
Inhibition of matrix *metalloproteinases*: a new *skin* care frontier. ...
To a large degree, the signs of *skin aging* reflect the condition of the *skin* matrix ...
www.smartskincare.com

Matrix *metalloproteinase*-1 and *skin aging* in smokers.
Lahmann C, Bergemann J, Harrison G, Young AR. Comment in: Lancet.
www.ncbi.nlm.nih.gov/pubmed/11289356

NEJM -- Pathophysiology of Premature *Skin Aging* Induced by...
Smoking and Skin Aging in Identical Twins. Arch Dermatol 143: 1543-1546 ... Matrix *Metalloproteinase* Expression in Normal *Skin* Associated with Basal Cell ...
content.nejm.org/cgi/content/short/337/20/1419

Sun ageing (again)

Improve Your *Skin* with Copper-Peptide Non Surgical *Skin*
Causes of *Skin Aging* - UV light, Detergents, Cortisone, Irritants.... of damaged and older *skin* by increasing the synthesis of metalloproteinases, Aging Reversal Sciences, *Skin* Biology, CP
www.skinbiology.com

Sun Damage to skin - How harmful is the sun
As time goes by and these *solar scars* are repeatedly damaged by the sun and as ... Not only are wrinkles and *solar scars* a result of UV damage from the suns ...
www.healthyskincream.com/sundamage

Journal of Investigative Dermatology - Topical N-Acetyl Cysteine
With each intermittent UV exposure, there is additional *solar scarring*, which alters the structural integrity of the dermis. ...
www.nature.com

Solar Scars | Age Spot | Looking For The Best Way To Prevent And
So not the same as age spots caused by a similar affliction I thought I'd take a minute to talk about *solar scars*. *Solar scars* are a formation
www.agespot-s.org/solar-scars

How smoking ages skin | Simply Anti Aging
After tanning - *smoking* is the worst thing you can do to your *skin*. *Smoking* causes wrinkles and gives you smokers face. Get the facts about *smoking* and *skin* ...
www.simplyantiaging.com/820/smoking-and-skin-aging

Causes of Aging Skin
Public knowledge, awareness, and perceptions of the association between *skin aging* and *smoking*." Journal of the American Academy
www.skincarephysicians.com/agingskinnet/basicfacts.html

Perfect *Skin* Dos and Don'ts
Here are 5 dos and 5 don'ts to help slowly down and reverse the *aging* process and leave your *skin* glowing at any age. Do stop *smoking*. Ever notice the *skin* of ...
beauty.about.com/od/skinflaws/a/agingskin.htm

BBC News | HEALTH | *Smoking* link to premature *aging*
Smoking destroys the ability of the *skin* to renew itself effectively, thus accelerating the *aging* process, a study has indicated.
news.bbc.co.uk/2/hi/health/710447.stm

Pollution

Tips - Microdermamitt | Direct Sales, Wholesale Exfoliating...
Although people may *have a genetic predisposition to severe wrinkling, particularly ozone,* may hasten aging by producing oxygen-free radicals. These are particles produced by many of the body's normal chemical processes; in excessive amounts they
www.microdermamitt.com

Wind damage

How to Protect _Skin_ From _Wind_ | eHow.com
Wind can _damage_ your _skin_ year-round, whether mixed with saltwater or snowflakes or during an otherwise normal sunny day. The _wind_ can leave your _skin_ dry,
www.ehow.com

Protecting Your _Skin_ from _Wind Damage_ - Associated Content
Will need to protect yourself against _skin damage_. _Skin_ doesn't just make you look pretty. It is also a barrier to disease and infection. ...
www.associatedcontent.com

How much does cold weather and _wind damage_ the _skin_?
I know how damaging the sun can be, but what about the cold. ... Yes, just as how extremely hot weather can _damage skin_, so can extremely cold
answers.yahoo.com/question/index?qid... - United States

Central heating skin dryness - Top Beauty Tips - Beauty Swap
Re: _Central heating skin_ dryness.... The sun is responsible for most of the _damage_ done to the _skin_. It causes dryness, wrinkles, and even rashes and ...
www.beautyswapshop.co.uk/Forum/tabid/54/.../2/.../Default.aspx

Skin problems | MaleHealth
Avoid overheating, as this increases _skin_ irritation. Turn down the _central heating_ and avoid overdressing or heavy bedcovers. ...
www.malehealth.co.uk/skin/18864-skin-problems

Eumovate Eczema and Dermatitis Cream for Itchy, Dry Skin Care...
Dry _skin_ is a major symptom of _skin_ flare-up and can also be part of the cause. ..Can create an allergic response or irritant chemicals that can cause damage. Central heating.
www.skinflare-up.com/prevention.asp

Skin care: winter-proof your _skin_
Save the planet as well as your _skin_ by turning the _central heating_ down a degree ..._damaging_ and drying effects of the cold weather and _central heating_. ...
www.ivillage.co.uk/.../skincare/.../0,,547687_183886-2,00.html

Sun Damage to Skin Causes Invisible as well as Visible Effects
Take this important first step to understand sun _damage to skin_. It can be as trivial as ...central heating and _air conditioning_. Hot showers or baths ...
www.1st-sunprotection-guide.com/sun-damage-to-skin.html

Skin Factors: Factors that affect Skin, Natural skin care factor
Air conditioning: If you spend long hours in an air-conditioned room or office, of skin. The damage is cumulative and may not be immediately apparent. ...
www.beauty-cosmetic-guide.com/skin-factors.htm

Essential Damage-care Hair Care « Beautyknot ~ My Skin Care
7 Jul 2010 ... Nuance Airy Damage Care Conditioner. (THB79/180ml, THB139/350ml) ... was particularly drying when I spent many hours in air-conditioning. ...
beautyknot.wordpress.com/2010/.../essential-damage-care-hair-care

Lax skin

Lax skin - definition of lax skin in the Medical dictionary - by...
Skin (skin) the outer protective covering of the body, consisting of the dermis (or corium) and the epidermis. Enlarge picture. Diagram of a cross-section ...
medical-dictionary.thefreedictionary.com/lax+skin

Lax Skin - WrongDiagnosis.com
List of 53 disease causes of Lax Skin, patient stories, diagnostic guides, medical books excerpts online about Lax Skin. Diagnostic checklist, medical tests ...
www.wrongdiagnosis.com

Lax Skin - Symptom Checker - check medical symptoms at Wrong
List of 42 causes of Lax Skin, alternative diagnoses, rare causes, misdiagnoses, patient stories, and much more.
symptoms.wrongdiagnosis.com/cosymptoms/lax-skin.htm

Occluded eyes

Retinal Vein Occlusion - Eye Help (UK)
Retinal vein occlusion occurs when the small veins that carry blood away from the retina become blocked. These blockages can be caused by blood clots ...
www.eyehelp.co.uk/retinal-vein-occlusion.html

Upper punctual *occlusion* versus lower punctual *occlusion* in dry *eye*
12 May 2010 ... There was no significant difference for any of these variables between upper punctum *occluded eyes* and lower punctum *occluded eyes* before or ...
www.iovs.org/cgi/content/abstract/iovs.09-5097v1

Retinal Vein *Occlusion*
Retinal vein *occlusion* is an *eye* condition commonly seen in most *eye* care offices. It is second only to diabetic retinopathy as a cause of visual loss due
www.avclinic.com/retinal_vein_occlusion.htm

Skin tags

Acrochordon - Wikipedia, the free encyclopedia
It is believed that *skin tags* occur from skin rubbing up against skin, there is now an over-the-counter solution that causes *skin tag* removal. ...
en.wikipedia.org/wiki/Acrochordon

Skin Tags, *Skin Tag* Removal and Treatment
Skin Tags - Compare the top 3 *skin tag* removal products to safely and effectively remove *skin tags* from the groin, face, armpits. Only at Skintaghelp.com.
www.skintaghelp.com

Skin Tags | Health | Embarrassing | Channel4.com/bodies
Skin tags are soft lumps, attached to the skin by a stalk that tends to occur in the armpits, neck and groins.
www.channel4embarrassingillnesses.com/conditions/skin-tags

Skin

Skin - Wikipedia, the free encyclopedia
3 In fish and amphibians; 4 In birds and reptiles; 5 See also This keratinized *layer* of *skin* is responsible for keeping water in the ... but other *types* of *skin* gland are found in other vertebrates. ... However,
en.wikipedia.org/wiki/Skin

Flashcards Table on A&P BIO 141: TISSUE *TYPES* AND S
Epithelium consisting of four *distinct* cell *types* and four or five *distinct layers*. It accounts for only 2-*3*% of *skin* cancers, but its incidence is ... Erythematic, pain, blistering, due to accumulation between *skin layers*. ...
www.proprofs.com/flashcards/tableview.php?...types

What are the three *layers* of *skin*-Education Questions answered
The *skin* is made up of three *distinct layers*. The top *layer* is called the epidermis. ... The dermis is composed of three *types* of tissue that are
www.qa02.com/edu/what-are-the-three-layers-of-skin.html

The epidermis
Each of these *types* has specific, and no less vital, functions. ... As they continuously slough off the surface of the *skin* in a process known as desquamation. 1 day. *3*.... On looking closely, two *distinct layers* of corneocytes can
www.skin-science.com/ .../topic_sousrub.aspx*?*

***Stratum corneum* - Wikipedia, the free encyclopedia**
From the Latin for horned layer, this *skin* layer is composed mainly of dead cells that lack nuclei. ... Replaced by new cells from the *stratum germinativum* (basale). ... Requiring the *palms* to be covered with a *thick stratum corneum*. ... In reptiles, the *stratum corneum* is
en.wikipedia.org/wiki/Stratum_corneum

***Stratum* - definition of *stratum* in the Medical dictionary - by the...**
The layer of epidermis between the stratum lucidum and stratum spinosum. 2. ... corneal layer. Stratum granulosum, n one of the layers of the epidermis or the ... only in the thick skin of the palms of the hands and the soles of the feet. ... 2. The deep layer of the cortex
medical-dictionary.thefreedictionary.com/stratum

Stratum lucidum: Definition from Answers.com
Stratum lucidum ('stradəm 'lüsədəm) (histology) A layer of irregular transparent ... only in the thick skin of the palms of the hands and the soles of the feet. ... Meaning #1: the layer of epidermis immediately under the stratum
www.answers.com/topic/clear-layer-of-epidermis

Skin Anatomy
Stratum Lucidum (present only in very thick skin); Stratum Granulosum (Granular ... (1) basal layer (stratum basale epidermidis); (2) spinous layer (stratum spinosum epidermidis); (3) granular layer (stratum granulosum epidermidis); (4) clear
www.fpnotebook.com/der/exam/sknantmy.htm

Anatomy Atlases: Atlas of Microscopic Anatomy: Section 7:
The epidermis of the palm and sole is thick (so-called thick skin) and has five ... From the deepest outward, the layers are (1) stratum basale, (2) stratum spinosum, (3) stratum granulosum, (4) stratum lucidum, and (5) stratum corneum. ... The stratum granulosumis
www.anatomyatlases.org/.../Section07/Section07.shtml

How can you distinguish between the *strata* of the epidermis in...?

16 Oct 2009 ... What would you *like* to ask? ... Located between the stratum granulosum and stratum corneum layers. ... *4.* The *stratum spinosum* (or spinous layer) is a layer of the... *5.* The *stratum germinativum* (or basal layer, *stratum* basale)
answers.yahoo.com

Stratum lucidum - wikidoc

18 Dec 2007 ... It is found beneath the *stratum corneum* of *thick skin*, such as that on the *palms* of the *hands* and the *soles* of ... Skin layers, cutis: Epidermis (*Stratum corneum, Stratum lucidum, Stratum granulosum, Stratum spinosum, Stratum* ... as well as an
www.wikidoc.org/index.php/Stratum_lucidum

Stratum germinativum

Stratum germinativum - Wikipedia, the free encyclopedia

The Stratum germinativum (or basal layer, stratum basale) is the deepest layer of the 5layers of the epidermis, which is the outer covering of skin in ...
en.wikipedia.org/wiki/Stratum_germinativum

Stratum germinativum - wikidoc

27 May 2008 ... Stratum germinativum (also stratum basale or basal cell layer) is the layer of ... Epidermis (skin) (5) · Stratum granulosum
www.wikidoc.org/index.php/Stratum_germinativum

Incorporation of 3H-thymidine in stratum germinativum of epidermi

In normal toads, the % of *stratum germinativum* cells that incorporated 3H-thymidine ... The skin of the thumb was dissected free, frozen rapidly in 2"5~o ...
linkinghub.elsevier.comThe Dermis

Dermis - Wikipedia, the free encyclopedia

The *dermis* is a *layer* of skin between the epidermis and subcutaneous tissues, and is composed of two *layers*, the *papillary* and *reticular dermis*. Structural ...
en.wikipedia.org/wiki/Dermis

Skin - Wikipedia, the free encyclopedia

Dermis. 2.2.1 *Papillary* region; 2.2.2 *Reticular* region ... This keratinized *layer* of skin is responsible for keeping water in the body and keeping other ...
en.wikipedia.org/wiki/Skin

Skin (Integumentary) System Information

The *papillary layer* lies directly beneath the epidermis and connects to ... The *reticular layer* of the *dermis* contains criss-crossing collagen ... glands secrete sweat, a mixture of 99 percent water and *1* percent salts and fats. ...
www.besthealth.com/besthealth/bodyguide/.../skin_sys_fin.html

Papillary *and* reticular dermal *fibroblasts - Biology Online*

30 Aug 2008 ... A vascular plexus, the rete subpapillare, demarcates the lower limit of the *papillary dermis* (Figs *1, 2*). The *reticular layer* of the *dermis* ...
www.biology-online.org

Skin - Anatomy - Skin *Layers*

9 Apr 2007 ... The two layers of the *dermis* are the papillary and *reticular layers.* The upper, *papillary layer*, contains a thin arrangement of collagen ...
dermatology.about.com

Reticular dermis
 The *reticular layer* of the *dermis* (RD) consists of dense irregular connective tissue, which h differs from the *papillary layer* (PD)
www.meddean.luc.edu

Skin (Integumentary) System Information
Jump to <u>Skin:</u> *dermal layers*: The *dermis* has two layers: the *papillary layer*, which has loose connective ... The *reticular layer* of the *dermis* contains...
www.besthealth.com

Dermis
The *reticular layer* is denser than the papillary *dermis*, and it strengthens the skin, providing structure and elasticity. It also supports other components ...
www.daviddarling.info

Definition of Papillary Layer | eHow.com
These are collagen, elastic and reticular fibers. While these are contained in both layers of the *dermis*, the *papillary layer* primarily has collagen fibers. ...
www.ehow.com

Ridges and Furrows - Development of Friction Skin
The *Dermis* is much thicker than the epidermis and consists of two layers - the *Papillary layer* (DPL) an area of loose connective tissue extending up into ...
ridgesandfurrows.homestead.com

Intergumentary system

Integumentary system - Wikipedia, the free encyclopedia
The *integumentary system* has a variety of *functions*; it may serve to waterproof, cushion
en.wikipedia.org/wiki/Integumentary system

Science Netlinks: The *Integumentary System*
The *integumentary system* has many *functions*, most of which are involved in protecting you and regulating your body's internal *functions* in a variety of ways ...
www.sciencenetlinks.com

Integumentary System Functions
The *integumentary system functions* consist of one of most important *functions* that are protecting delicate inner parts of body from infection, dust, etc.
www.buzzle.com

Apoptosis

Chapter 9: Cell Death, *Including Apoptosis* - Flow Cytometry
1 Apr 2010 ... Chapter 9: Cell Death, *Including Apoptosis* ... Before commencing any study of apoptosis using flow cytometry, you should, whenever possible,
flowbook-wiki.denovosoftware.com

Study *including apoptosis*. Ticlopidine induced colitis: a...
Study *including apoptosis*. D Berrebi, A Sautet, J-F Flejou, M-C Dauge, M Peuchmaur, F Potet. Abstract. Aims—To describe ticlopidine related mi- ...
jcp.bmj.com/content/51/4/280.full.pdf

Cell Death and Differentiation - Terminal differentiation of human...
Interestingly, some features of *terminally differentiating keratinocytes* resemble cellular changes associated with apoptosis. This implies that classical ...
www.nature.com

Human *keratinocytes* that have not terminally differentiated
Human *keratinocytes* that have not *terminally differentiated* synthesize laminin and fibronectin but deposit only fibronectin in the pericellular matrix. ...
www.ncbi.nlm.nih.gov/pubmed/2416765

Thermoregulation

Thermoregulation - Wikipedia, the free encyclopedia
Thermoregulation is the ability of an organism to keep its body temperature within certain boundaries, even when the surrounding temperature is very ...
en.wikipedia.org/wiki/Thermoregulation

Temperature Homeostasis (thermoregulation)
In humans, body temperature is controlled by the *thermoregulatory* centre in the ... It is only when these responses are not enough that the *thermoregulatory* ...
www.biologymad.com

Dictionary - Definition of *thermoregulation*
Thermoregulation is the ability of an organism to keep its body temperature within certain boundaries, even when temperature surrounding is very different. ...
www.websters-online-dictionary.org/th

Vitamen D

Vitamin D: Production, Metabolism, and Mechanisms of Action
1, 25(OH)2D is the principal hormonal form of *vitamin D*, responsible for most of its biologic actions. The *production* of 1, 25(OH) 2D in the kidney is tightly ...
www.endotext.org/parathyroid

Vitamin D
Many *vitamin D* supplements also contain high contents of vitamin A - and recent ... 25-OH-*Vitamin D*. 1, 25 (OH)2-*Vitamin D*. Liver. Kidney. Skin *production* ...
Courses.washington.edu/bonephys/opvitD.html

Vitamin D - Human skin production of vitamin D
A selection of articles related to Vitamin D - Human skin *production of vitamin D*.
www.experiencefestival.com/vitamin_d

Wound healing

Mast cells have been studied from a micro-chemical *stand*- point by.
Mast cells clearly Granules faintly defined and with stained purple to distinctly red; rapidly losing tendency. Their color on *stand*- ...
www.ncbi.nlm.nih.gov/pmc/articles

Identification of mast cells in the scanning
The two *mast cells stand* out with particular clarity. The unidentified large cell does not. (Stereos can. x 1000). Tilt angle = 33°.) FIGURE
jcb.rupress.org/cgi/reprint/61/3/641.pdf

Bone Marrow-derived *Mast Cell* - What does BMMC *stand* for?
Acronym, Definition. BMMC, Bone Marrow-derived *Mast Cell*. BMMC, British Motorsport Marshals
Club. BMMC, Bishkek Migration Management Center (Kyrgyz Republic ...
acronyms.thefreedictionary.com/Bone+Marrow-derived+Mast+Cell

The Epidermis

Keratin cytoskeletons in *epithelial cells* of internal organs — PNAS
When primary cultures of *epithelial cells* derived from bladder, intestine, kidney, and trachea were
grown on glass cover slips and stained with anti-*keratin*,
www.pnas.org/content/76/6/2813.short

Cytokeratin - Wikipedia, the free encyclopedia
Keratin intermediate filaments in *epithelial cells* (red stain the subsets of cytokeratins which
an *epithelial cell* expresses depends mainly on the.
en.wikipedia.org/wiki/Cytokeratin

Keratin - Wikipedia, the free encyclopedia
During the process of *epithelial* differentiation, *cells* become cornified as *keratin* protein is
incorporated into longer *keratin* intermediate filaments. ...
en.wikipedia.org/wiki/Keratin

Stratum corneum

Stratum Corneum Anatomy - Desquamation Process
The desquamation, or *exfoliation*, process of the *stratum corneum* is actually very complex and
only parts of this process are fully understood.
dermatology.about.com/od/anatomy/ss/sc_anatomy_9.htm

Topical Vitamin C for Beautiful Skin Without *Exfoliation*
27 Jun 2010 ... The thinning of this layer, known as the *stratum corneum* ... that *exfoliation* so often
does, but it works not by *gradually* wearing away the ...
mergemedia.com

Keratinocyte - definition of keratinocyte in the Medical
The granular cell layer, in which the cells become flattened and slowly die to form the final layer,
the stratum corneum, which gradually exfoliates
medical-dictionary.thefreedictionary.com/keratinocyte

Buy Dermalogica Products Online, Skin Care Logic Spa Dallas TX...
Ultimately reach your *stratum corneum* (the outermost layer of your skin) where ... It is possible to
over-*exfoliate*! Thicker skin can typically handle more ... per week...if you skin reacts favorably, feel
free to *gradually* add a day. ...
www.skincarelogic.com/exfoliation.htm -

Cornfied

Top Layer of the Epidermis - Stratum Corneum Anatomy -
The stratum corneum is the outermost of the 5 layers of the epidermis and is largely responsible for
the vital barrier function of the skin.
dermatology.about.com/od/anatomy/ss/sc_anatomy_5.htm –

Cornified - Wiktionary
13 Sep 2009 ... cornified (comparative more cornified, superlative most cornified) ... The least cornified, young cells stain violet or blue
en.wiktionary.org/wiki/cornified

Cornified - definition of cornified in the Medical dictionary
Converted into horny tissue (keratin); keratinized. How to thank TFD for its existence? Tell a friend about us, add a link to this page, add the site to ...
medical-dictionary.thefreedictionary.com/cornified

Stratum lucidum

Stratum lucidum - Wikipedia, the free encyclopedia
The stratum lucidum is a layer of the epidermis found throughout the body, but is thickest on the palms of the hands and the soles of the
en.wikipedia.org/wiki/Stratum_lucidum

Tapetum lucidum - Wikipedia, the free encyclopedia
The tapetum lucidum (Latin: "bright tapestry", plural tapeta lucida) is a layer of tissue in the eye of many vertebrate animals, that lies
en.wikipedia.org/wiki/Tapetum_lucidum

Stratum germinativum - Wikipedia, the free encyclopedia
The Stratum germinativum (or basal layer, stratum basale) is the deepest layer of the 5 layers of the epidermis, which is the outer covering of skin in ...
en.wikipedia.org/wiki/Stratum_germinativum

Stratum germinativum
The stratum germinatum (SG) provides the germinal cells necessary for the regeneration of the layers of the epidermis. ...
www.meddean.luc.edu/lumen/MedEd/medicine/.../stgerm.htm

Stratum germinativum: Definition from Answers.com
Stratum germinativum ('stradəm 'jərmənə'tīvəm) (histology) The innermost germinative layer of
www.answers.com/topic/stratum-germinativum-1

Melanin - Wikipedia, the free encyclopedia
Dermal melanin is produced by melanocytes, which are found in the stratum basale of the epidermis. Although human beings generally possess a similar
en.wikipedia.org/wiki/Melanin

Effect of macrophages on elimination of dermal melanin from the
rophages in the elimination of dermal melanin in incontinentia pigmenti. H. Takematsu and M. Seiji: Elimination of Dermal
www.springerlink.com/index/LVQ73772530MM202.pdf

SIAscopy assists in the diagnosis of melanoma by utilizing ...
Information on the depth of melanin within the papillary dermis can also be.... Such structures can be clearly seen by examining the dermal melanin ...
events.cs.bham.ac.uk/miua2001/papers/Moncrieff

Definition of Papillary Layer | eHow.com
Definition of Papillary *Layer*. The skin of the human body is its most extensive organ system. It is the primary line of defense against disease causing ...
www.ehow.com

260

Skin (Integumentary) System Information
Jump to Skin: Dermal *layers*. The dermis has two layers: the *papillary layer*, which has loose connective ... The *reticular layer* of the dermis, contains ...
www.besthealth.com/
Reticular dermis

Reticular dermis
The *reticular layer of the dermis* (RD) consists of dense irregular connective tissue, which differs from the papillary layer (PD),
www.meddean.luc.edu

Skin - Anatomy - Skin *Layers*
9 Apr 2007 ... The two layers of the dermis are the papillary and reticular layers. The upper, *papillary layer*, contains a thin arrangement of collagen ...
dermatology.about.com/c

Skin (Integumentary) System Information
Jump to Skin: dermal layers. The dermis has two layers: the papillary layer, which has loose connective ... The reticular layer of the dermis contains ...
www.besthealth.com/besthealth/body

Langer's lines

Langer's lines,
Sometimes called cleavage lines, are topological lines drawn on a map of the human body. They technically are defined by the direction
en.wikipedia.org/wiki/Langer's_lines

Langer's lines *of the skin*
Langer's lines, also called cleavage lines, is a term used to define the direction within the human skin along which the skin has the least
www.med-ars.it/galleries/langer.htm

Netter Medical Artwork - *Langer's Lines*
Rights-managed illustration with leader lines and labels of *Langer's Lines* from the Netter Collection, drawn by Carlos AG Machado.
www.netterimages.com/image/7446.htm

COLLAGEN GUIDE *Collagen* **information Products**
The only thing better would be to *take* a bio-available *collagen* supplement directly. ... When *collagen* disease strikes *as we age*, this shock absorbing quality is reduced. ... To the body's lack of *collagen* and its ongoing *collagen*
www.sesderma.co.uk/collagen.htm

Genacol and *Collagen* **Diseases - The Key to Youth, page 1**
Early on, our hands start to take on the wrinkled dishpan look so ... a selective *destructive* of *collagen* in the joint cartilage has occurred. That much of the body's vital metabolic repair work takes place when we sleep. ... When *collagen* disease
www.1234yourhealth.com/Collagen_Key_Youth_01.htm

Destruction of Collagen in our Skin Causes Fine Lines and Wrinkles
11 Jan 2009 .As we age the effectiveness of the protein that forms *collagen*. Do you know what?
www.articlesbase.com

Skin Aging & Wrinkles: Dealing with Sun Damage & Collagen
For example, while we know that *collagen* and elastin, ... It would *take* an entire book to evaluate every element of the skin affected by intrinsic ... but it is important to get a basic sense of what is taking *place* to better ... Furthermore, for some unknown reason,
www.cosmeticscop.com

Exercise Increases Collagen
11 Sep 2009 ... Exercise Increases Collagen*; Ibuprofen Inhibits This Effect* ... stresses of exercise activate a particular molecular pathway that increases ...
houseofverona.com/exercise-increases-collagen

Cortisol - Wikipedia, the free encyclopedia
However cortisol *increases* glycogen synthesis (glycogenesis) in the liver. An enzyme which is used to cross link *collagen* and elastin. ..Because of its *molecular* similarity to aldosterone, it also binds to the ..."Cortisol responses to mental *stress, exercise,*
en.wikipedia.org/wiki/Cortisol

How to *Build* Collagen and *Elastin*
8 Feb 2010 ... Have you ever wondered how to *build* collagen and *elastin* that will tighten your skin naturally? Even when a dermatologist tells you that it ...
ezinearticles.com/?How-to-Build-Collagen-and-Elastin&id

Enterex® Diabetic Product & Nutrition Facts
Works with Zinc and Vitamin C to *build elastin*, an important skin protein.
Copper is important in healing, energy production, and taste sensitivity and is ...
www.enterexdiabetic.com/nut_facts.htm

Natural Skincare Ingredients Can Re-*Build* Collagen And *Elastin*
13 Feb 2009 ... When was the last time you bought a skin care product? Did you buy your regular brand just like you always do, or were you tempted to find ...
www.articlealley.com

Can Elastin Be Absorbed Into The Skin? - No!
29 Sep 2009 ... If not -- you may like to visit my website below, to learn more about how to naturally *build elastin* and collagen protein

www.articlesbase.com/.../can-elastin-be-absorbed-into-the-skin-no

What are free radicals*?*
Normally, the body can handle free radicals, but if antioxidants are unavailable, or if the free-radical production becomes excessive, damage can occur. ...
www.healthy-vitamin-choice.com/free-radicals.html

Understanding *Free Radicals* and Antioxidants
Normally, the body can handle free radicals, but if antioxidants are unavailable, or if the free-radical production becomes excessive, damage can occur. ...
www.healthchecksystems.com/antioxid.htm

Free radicals and your health
When cells in the *body* encounter a *free radical*, the reactive radical may ... another name for the chemical reaction that *free radicals* cause, *can* lead to a ...
www.healingdaily.com/conditions/free-radicals.htm

Antioxidants and *Free radicals*

To prevent *free radical* damage the *body* has a defense system of antioxidants. Antioxidants are molecules which *can* safely interact with *free radicals* and ...

www.rice.edu/~jenky/sports/antiox.html

Oxygen and the *Skin*

O2 Renew also assists with increasing the moisture content of the *skin* by increasing the *oxygen* level. O2 Renew also *does* not clog *skin* pores, nor interfere ...

www.o2renewsystem.com/oxygenandtheskin.htm

Does my skin need extra *oxygen*?

14 Sep 2009 ... Skin Actives (Official Rep) asked this question September

getsatisfaction.com/skinactives

Skin Care Products - neaclear Liquid *Oxygen Skin* Care Products

How *does oxygen* benefit acne-prone *skin*? *Oxygen* helps to heal acne and acne-prone *skin* types by reducing the number of acne-producing bacteria on the *skin's* ...

www.neaclear.com/faqs.shtml

Smoking Cessation - WHAT SMOKING *DOES* TO YOUR BODY

Smoking constricts the blood vessels in your *skin*, decreasing the delivery ... Because carbon monoxide lowers your blood *oxygen* carrying capacity; the blood ... nicotine in tobacco smoke increases the heart

www.smoking-cessation.org/content/healthissues.asp

How to Use *Oxygen* to Improve *Skin* | eHow.com

Introducing *oxygen* to the *skin* will give your face a clearer and refreshed look. ... EHow Terms of Use † and Privacy Policy †. en-US † *requires* javascript ...

www.ehow.com

Anti-, Tips, Staying Young, Herbs, Teas, Food for Aging, Life ...

It also *decreases* the conditions of angina pectoris and palpitation. ..... Mental and physical stamina, reducing muscle fatigue and *neutralizes free radicals*. ..... This *inflammation* process is due to an excess of *free radicals* which ... most

 www.peacefulmind.com/anti-aging.htm

Ag3derm | *Age Spots*, Liver Spots & Keratosis Totally Removed

Age spots, liver spots & keratosis treatment at home in 14 days. Watch it happen on video. Seborrheic keratosis & Actinic keratosis.

www.ag3derm.com/

Age Spots Home Remedy

Find *age spots* treatments and home remedies for *age spots* and sun spots, using natural cures and herbal products.

www.homeremediesweb.com/age_spots_home_remedy.php

What are *Age Spots*?

Brief and Straightforward Guide: What are *Age Spots*?

www.wisegeek.com/what-are-age-spots.htm

Liver *spot* - Wikipedia, the free encyclopedia

Liver spots (also known as "Solar lentigo", "Lentigo senilis" :686, "Old *age spot*," "Senile freckle") are blemishes on the skin associated with aging and ...

en.wikipedia.org/wiki/Liver spot

Collagen Skin Repair - This Will Help Rejuvenate Your Skin
21 May 2010 ... For people in their late 30's, collagen skin repair is an old-age favorite ... to lose it youthful juices resulting to uncontrolled increase.
ezinearticles.com/?Collagen-Skin-Repair...Rejuvenate

Adding To The Rejuvenation And Elasticity Of Skin
In Addition to the skin, collagen proteins can be found in the bones and ... I was able to repair the damage to my knees and once again walk without pain. ... To increase or decrease the amount of life affirming hydrolyzed collagen I ...
hubpages.com

Facial Treatments For Wrinkles
Perfector will lift sagging muscles and increase collagen, elastin and ... This process rejuvenates the skin, giving it a more firm and younger appearance. and antioxidant green tea is Pevonia Power
www.anti-aging-skin-care-guide.com/facial-treatmentsorwrinkles.html

Temporomandibular joint syndrome

Temporomandibular joint - Wikipedia, the free encyclopedia
Formation of the TMJ occurs at around 12 weeks in uterus when the joint ... by an articular disc, which divides the TMJ into two distinct compartments. ...
en.wikipedia.org/wiki/Temporomandibular_joint

Temporomandibular Joint (TMJ) Disorder Exercises, Surgery...
Temporomandibular joint (TMJ) syndrome is pain in the jaw joint that can be caused by a variety of medical problems. The TMJ connects the lower jaw ...
www.emedicinehealth.com

TMJ disorders - MayoClinic.com
TMJ disorders — Comprehensive overview covers symptoms and treatment, including, surgery.
www.mayoclinic.com/health/tmj-disorders/ds00355

Isometric Exercise

Isometric exercise - Wikipedia, the free encyclopedia
Isometric exercise or isometrics are a type of strength training in which the joint angle and muscle length do not change during contraction (compared to ...
en.wikipedia.org/wiki/Isometric_exercise

Isometric Exercises: How to Strengthen Abs, Legs, and Shoulders
Isometric exercise is a form of resistance training in which the participant uses the muscles of the body to exert a force either against an immovable ...
www.howtodothings.com/.../a3974-how-to-do-isometric-exercises

Isometric Exercise
Isometric exercise is practiced by pushing or pulling an immovable object like a wall or bar anchored to the floor. Research has shown that a muscle ...
www.questformuscle.com/articles/isometric-exercise

Dynamic Exercise

Dynamic Vs. Static Exercise: Health Topics: University of Iowa...
Dynamic exercise activities keep joints and muscles moving. Examples are swimming, walking, cross country skiing, bicycling, weight training,
www.uihealthcare.com/topics/exercisefitness/exer4494

Dynamic Stretching and Mobility Exercises
Examples of dynamic stretching and mobility exercises, which could form part of the warm up program in your training session.
www.brianmac.co.uk/dynamic

Isometric exercise - Wikipedia, the free encyclopedia
Isometric exercises have some differences in training effect as compared to dynamic exercises. While isometric training increases strength at the specific...
en.wikipedia.org/wiki/Isometric exercise

Isotonic Exercise

Isometric exercise - Wikipedia, the free encyclopedia
Isometric exercises are often made into parts of normal, **isotonic** exercises. ... Journal of applied physiology: respiratory,
en.wikipedia.org/wiki/Isometric exercise

Definitions of isotonic (exercise physiology)
Synonyms, antonyms, derivatives of isotonic (exercise physiology), analogical
dictionary.sensagent.com/isotonic+ (exercise physiology)/en-en

Isotonic (exercise physiology)
Isotonic (exercise physiology). In an isotonic contraction, tension rises and the skeletal muscle's length changes. Lifting an object off a desk, walking,
www.worldlingo.com/ma/enwiki/en/Isotonic_ (exercise_physiology)

Chapter 4

Celebrity Images

Sigourney Weaver | Showbiz Spy - celebrity news, rumors & gossip
DON'T expect to see Sigourney Weaver booking a consultation with her plastic surgeon. The Avatar star, 60, thinks cosmetic procedures are unnatural — and ...
www.showbizspy.com

A 360 report for Sigourney Weaver rumors
11 Jul 2010 ... DON'T expect to see Sigourney Weaver booking a consultation with her plastic surgeon. The Avatar star, 60, thinks cosmetic procedures are ...
www.360reports.com/demo.php?sterm=Sigourney+Weaver

Why 60 is the new 40 - Dear Miriam - Mirror.co.uk
26 Jan 2010 ... Even top stars once felt written off after 35 - but at 60, Sigourney Weaver has a big new hit in Avatar and her ... Here are just a few things that those clocking up the years can feel smug about. ... These days, a healthy 60-year-old woman can expect another 20 to 30 mostly
blogs.mirror.co.uk/dear-miriam/.../why-60-is-the-new-40.html

Female celebrities and plastic surgery | Simply Anti Aging
Fonda – now in her 70's – said she would prefer to age gracefully and not ... Still young looking Andie MacDowell – from a slightly younger generation than Bisset or Fonda – has also been quite forthright in her views against plastic surgery ... in a good
www.simplyantiaging.com

Andie MacDowell anti aging without plastic surgery
Andie MacDowell manages to be an anti aging icon without plastic surgery - but ...Andie MacDowell has stayed looking younger than her true age of 50 and what's more she is on record as saying she definitely doesn't believe in plastic surgery. ... MacDowell
www.simplyantiaging.com

LIZ JONES: It's never been easier to look fabulous at 50, all you
29 May 2009 ... Model - actress Andie MacDowell attends the 7th Annual 'Dressed to Kilt'... my generation, has such a different attitude towards aging is.... Botox alone wouldn't account for their good looks - diet, exercise, good skin care, and its only
www.dailymail.co.uk

Female celebrities and plastic surgery | Simply Anti Aging
Despite this several high profile young celebrities have spoken out against surgery including: Kate Winslet, Kate Beckinsale and Diane
www.simplyantiaging.com

KATE WINSLET BIOGRAPHY
Female celebrities and plastic surgery | Simply Anti Aging. Despite this several high profile young celebrities have spoken out against surgery including: Kate Winslet, Kate Beckinsale and
www.simplyantiaging.com

Celebrity Cosmetic Surgery:
The Premiere Site For Celebrity Plastic Surgery By A Real Plastic Surgeon ... Diane Lane is adamant she will grow old without the aid of cosmetic surgery.... site to Awful Plastic Surgery) is reporting that Kate Beckinsale may have had .... A young woman from
celebritycosmeticsurgery.blogspot.com

My Lot - Diane Lane is The New Face of Neutrogena
On Friday, November 16th, Diane Lane has signed on to be the ambassador for Neutrogena, which is worldwide leader in the development of highly...
www.mylot.com/w/blogarticle/529292.aspx

Beauty Byte: Diane Lane Is the New Face of Neutrogena
16 Nov 2007 ... This just in: Diane Lane has become a "brand ambassador" for Neutrogena. Like Jennifer Garner, she'll appear in advertisements for the ...
www.bellasugar.com

Nose Jobs (rhinoplasty) | In Your Face
I am hesitant to write about someone who died so recently," he said. ... Shields haven't admitted having plastic surgery, but she has often been subject of .year, as In Your Face reported, Shields said she was undecided whether she would have. Plastic surgeon Dr.
inyourface.ocregister.com/tag/nose-job-rhinoplasty

OH NO, THEY DIDN'T.
25 Jan 2010 ... She said the former "Beautiful Life" actress is "an amazing professional, lovely to work with. Lynch, a 49-year-old native of Dolton, Illinois, has carved out ... But then I wonder how these people know I have a gay following Tila admits to her own
community.livejournal.com/ohnotheydidnt/2010/01/25

Female celebrities and plastic surgery | Simply Anti Aging
Jane Seymour takes a similar line despite admitting to having had plastic surgery to reduce the bags under her eyes. The British actress who is in her 50's has said she is against plastic...Interestingly there seems to be more tolerance of plastic surgery among
www.simplyantiaging.com

Celebrity Cosmetic Surgery: Jane Seymour Admits to Plastic Surgery
56 Year old Actress Jane Seymour has recently admitted to having plastic surgery. ... The bags"), breast implants (so small her plastic surgeon had to ... It's refreshing to see a star like her admit to well-done plastic surgery. ... Jane looks
celebritycosmeticsurgery.blogspot.com

Seymour, Jane - Make Me Heal
24 Feb 2009 ... British actress Jane Seymour's 26-year old daughter Katie looks like she could be a ... Moreover, it appears she had a few other cosmetic surgery ... Seymour has no plans to go under the knife in the near future and has ... "I've
education.makemeheal.com/index.php/Seymour, Jane

Chapter 5

Facial Surgery and Alternatives

Why does this chapter have so many references?
Simple, because I have done my homework for you!

If I could find a cream, gadget or something that actually worked I could stop doing facial exercises. Would I use it? Yes, to be perfectly honest. Fitface is like going to the gym I would prefer to be lazy, forego the natural high and accomplishment and slap on a cream each morning and look 10 years younger! But it isn't available!

Face-lifts & cosmetic surgery

Stem Cell Facelift
Cutting edge Non-Surgical Facelift Top Cosmetic Physician
www.BodyCareDoctor.com

Facelift - Guide to Face Lift Surgery - Risks, Cost & Benefits
They are often used in conjunction with facelift plastic surgery. ... A thread lift is not the same as a facelift, but it is a cosmetic facial procedure What Does a Facelift Cost - Thread Lift - Eyelid surgery -
www.yourplasticsurgeryguide.com/face-lift

A Natural Face Lift and Neck Lift-
FaceLift, Macs Face Lift, Mid Face Lift, Mini Face Lift, Endoscopic Face Lift, Feather Lift, Thread Face Lift, Subperiosteal Face Lift, QuickLift, S Face ... I like the Temporal Mid - Face / Cheek Lift
www.cosmeticsurg.com/thousand_oaks_face_lift.html

Endotine Bioabsorbable Implant by Coapt Systems, -
The Thread Face Lift another procedure for lifting the cheek and Mid-Face area cannot create the same effect as the ... Face Lift, Macs Face Lift, Mid Face Lift, Mini Face Lift, Endoscopic Face Lift, Feather Lift, Thread Face Lift, Subperiosteal Face Lift, Quick lift, S Face Lift,
www.cosmeticsurg.com

Lifestyle Lift Procedure Problems | eHow.com
Lifestyle Lift Procedure Problems. As we age our facial skin tends to sag and wrinkle. ...These surgeries run the gamut from relatively simple eyelid lifts to ... The mini facelift procedure has
www.ehow.com

Non Surgical Feather Lift Procedures | eHow.com
How to Get a Non Surgical Face Lift with the Galvanic Spa ... Difference Between Smas Facelift & Lifestyle Facelift; Can You Use Botox If You've Had ... The quickness of this procedure has earned it the name, "lunch time face lift." The lure of this procedure is that
www.ehow.com

Your thoughts on Ribbon lift? Doctor answers on RealSelf.com
What's the latest thought on ribbon lifts? Things move on so quickly, A full, comprehensive face/neck lift addresses excess fat in the neck, catchy phrases "ribbon", "lunchtime", "thread"
www.realself.com

Doctor Linda Huang - Face Procedures
But realistically, none can be done over the lunch break and have you back at work by three.... First, then, the mini-lift, lifestyle lift, quick lift and MACS–lift (minimal ... I have been having a lot of fun with these little lifts lately. ... A neck lift is usually combined with
www.lindahuangmd.com/pro-face.html

Lifestyle Lift®
Safe, Effective, Low-Cost Lifts-- Contact Today To Look Years Younger
www.LifestyleLift.com

Face Lifts Procedures
Ask.com/Face-Lifts

Textbook for General and Oral Surgery
It has a straight blade and is designed to lift the epiglottis anteriorly displacement of all mid-face fractures tends to be downwards and. These separations have allowed the face to be divided
www.scribd.com

Browplasty

Brow Lift | Forehead Lift | Browplasty | Cosmetic Surgery Today
Other terms associated with Forehead Lift Surgery: Brow Lift, Browplasty. Brow lift Overview: A forehead lift, also commonly referred to as both a brow lift and a ... Multiple surgical approaches can be utilized in forehead lift procedures. ... Lift only
www.cosmeticsurgerytoday.com/brow-lift

Los Angeles Brow lift Surgery – Brow lifts in Beverly Hills, CA
Endoscopic brow elevation is the most current and state-of-the art method of... In the past decade, the endoscopic forehead and brow lift has rapidly become Botulinum toxin may be used
www.spaldingplasticsurgery.com/procedures_browlift.html

Blepharoplasty

Meronk - Eyebrow Surgery
Direct brow lift, in which the incision is made just above the eyebrow hair ... the brow is stabilized through the upper blepharoplasty incision (see photo links below) ...Cable brow lift, in which thick suture placed deep below the skin ... A brow or forehead lift (coronal or
www.drmeronk.com/insidersguide/16.html

Direct brow lift - Review of Ophthalmology
Variations in supraciliary direct brow lift incisions. ... Since the mid-forehead lift results in tightening of the skin, wrinkles that ... The supraciliary incision is created just within the uppermost hair of the brow to best hide. A standard blepharoplasty incision is created
www.revophth.com/index.asp

Browplasty: Treatment – e Medicine Otolaryngology and Facial...

Because the incisions are placed relatively close to the brow, asymmetry is... The upper blepharoplasty incision is used to access the forehead wrinkles, brow wrinkles, and facial aesthetic
emedicine.medscape.com

Comprehensive Management of Eyebrow and Forehead Ptosis

Traditionally, this has been accomplished through a direct eyebrow lift approach. The incision is placed in a rhytid 1 to 1.5 cm above the brow. The depth of the incision is just posterior under the subcutaneous fat. A blepharoplasty incision is made and blunts
linkinghub.elsevier.com/retrieve/pii/S0030666505000721

Selling dreams

CBC News - Health - Quebec doctors clamp down on cosmetic surgery

Jun 15, 2010. "It looks like we sell dreams," said Lamontagne. Ontario doctors tighten cosmetic surgery regulations · Cosmetic surgery lures away ...
www.cbc.ca/health/story/.../mtl-college-of-physicians-cosmetic-surgery.html

Wichita – Heartland Cosmetic and Reconstructive Surgery

Heartland Cosmetic Surgery and Salina Surgical Arts Center is proud to announce the ...Heartland Dr. David Hendrick is helping people realize their dreams. ...
www.heartlandcosmeticsurgery.com/

Wind tunnel effect

Facelift Tampa *Face Lift* St Petersburg Rhytidectomy Clearwater

If the skin or muscles are pulled too much in their line of pull then the "*wind tunnel*" *effect* can occur. Not all traditional *face lifts* result in
www.egoziplasticsurgery.com/face-lift.htm

Facelifts

However, we have all seen people who have had "extreme" *facelifts*, with the "wind-tunnel" effect on their skin. It is our belief that simple facelifts get ...
www.dryoho.com/dr-yoho-book/chapter8-1.cfm

Creams & Cosmeceuticals

Cosmeceuticals - Wikipedia, the free encyclopedia

Cosmeceuticals represent the marriage of cosmetics and pharmaceuticals. Examples of products typically labeled as *Cosmeceuticals* include anti-aging creams ...
en.wikipedia.org/wiki/Cosmeceuticals

Perricone MD - Skin Care Products, *Cosmeceuticals* & Prescription

Official site of Perricone MD for bestselling anti-aging *Cosmeceuticals*, anti-inflammatory diet, skin care supplements, and acne treatments.
www.perriconemd.com

Cosmeceuticals: eMedicine Dermatology

Jun 22, 2010. Overview: *Cosmeceuticals* represent a marriage between cosmetics and pharmaceuticals. Like cosmetics, *Cosmeceuticals* are topically applied
emedicine.medscape.com

Cosmeceuticals
Because *Cosmeceuticals* are not subject to approval by the U.S. Food and Drug Administration ... The new trend in *Cosmeceuticals* is combination products. ...
www.aad.org/media/background/.../fact_cosmeceuticals.html

Cosmeceuticals Facts & Your Skin
Cosmeceuticals Facts pamphlet Cosmetics are used to color and adorn the body in a ....*Cosmeceuticals*, colored cosmetics, and skin care products are part of ...
www.aad.org/public/publications/.../general_cosmeceutical.html

Cosmeceuticals
Because *Cosmeceuticals* are not subject to approval by the U.S. Food and Drug Administration ... The new trend in *Cosmeceuticals* is combination products. ...
www.aad.org/media/background/.../fact_cosmeceuticals.html

Sircuit Cosmeceuticals
Offers a new line of Natural Skin Care Products designed to combat the visible effects of aging by restoring and maintaining
www.sircuitskin.com

What Are Cosmeceuticals? Sep 19, 2009
Cosmeceuticals straddle the line between cosmetics and drugs
www.webmd.com/skin-beauty

Skin Wrinkles
Tretinoin (known commercially as Retin-A) is the only topical agent approved for treating ....Alpha Hydroxy acids facilitate the shedding of dead skin cells and may even stimulate ...Prescription strength creams contain at least 12% glycolic acid, ... Response t
adam.about.com/reports/000021

Retinol vs Alpha Hydroxy Acid vs Glycolic Acid
Staples: Glycolic acid cleanser, Skin Ceuticals Phloretin CF, Revaleskin, NIA24. ... Other retinol products are using a different A) is the gold standard for anti-aging... I'd previously been prescribed
www.essentialdayspa.com/forum/viewthread.php?tid

Safe skin care during pregnancy | BabyCenter
Some studies have shown that high doses of vitamin A during pregnancy can be harmful to an ... Retin-A, Renova (tretinoin) Retinoic acid. Retinol Retinyl linoleate. Note: Alpha hydroxy acids, sometimes listed as AHAs, glycolic acid was on ORAL ingestion of
www.babycenter.com

Hydroquinone

Hydroquinone Is Dangerous
Learn Which Creams Use Hydroquinone Find Out Before You Buy!
Skin-Treatment-Association.com

Stop Using Hydroquinone
Lighten Skin without Dangerous Hydroquinone. Avoid Side Effects
CivantSkinCare.com/Hydroquinone

Hydroquinone - Wikipedia, the free encyclopedia
Hydroquinone, also benzene-1, 4-diol or quinol, is an aromatic organic compound which is a type of phenol, having the chemical formula $C_6H_4(OH)_2$
en.wikipedia.org/wiki/Hydroquinone

Vit E
Quality Vitamin E, Buy 1 Get 2 Free 100% Freshness, Purity & Potency
www.Puritan.com

Information on Vitamin E
Picking a Vitamin Can be Confusing. Make the Right Choice at AOL Health
www.AOLhealth.com

Vitamin E
Dec 15, 2009. Vitamin E is found naturally in some foods, added to others, and available as a
dietary supplement. "Vitamin E" is the collective name for a.
ods.od.nih.gov/factsheets/vitamine.asp

Vitamin E - Wikipedia, the free encyclopedia
Vitamin E is a generic term for tocopherols and tocotrienols.
Vitamin E is a family of α-, β-, γ-, and δ- (respectively: alpha, beta
en.wikipedia.org/wiki/Vitamin E

Vitamin C

Vitamin C serum | Skin Care
I recommend everyone put Vitamin C and E onto their face daily because they ... is a risk that
before you get your precious vitamin C cream or serum home,
www.natural-skin-care-info.com/vitamin-c-serum.html

Can a cream make you look younger?
May 23, 2007 ... Vitamin C is an antioxidant that can lighten pigment, and is one of the most
popular constituents in products today. But in cream form,
www.netdoctor.co.uk/womenshealth/features/miracle.htm

Vitamin C Cream -
Vitamin C Cream - 660 results like the Botanic Choice Vitamin C Cream, Avalon Organic Vitamin
C Renewal Facial Cream -- 2 oz, Emergin C vitamin c cream
www.nextag.com/vitamin-c-cream/stores-html

Facial Moisturizers: Best Face Moisturizer Reviews
America Rx.c- om AmericaRx.com for $20.22 · Amazon... If you have sensitive skin,
reviews recommend Aveeno Ultra-Calming Daily Moisturizer SPF 15. ... Skin Anti-Wrinkle Cream,
which contains retinol, a vitamin A derivative
www.consumersearch.com/moisturizers

Alpha Lipoic Acid

Lipoic acid - Wikipedia, the free encyclopedia
Lipoic Acid Biosynthesis. Chapter 2 in in Alpha Lipoic Acid: Energy the Urinary Excretion and
Serum level of Alpha Lipoic Acid in
wikipedia.org/wiki/Lipoic acid

Alpha Lipoic Acid (ALA) | Alpha Lipoic Acid Benefits and Side Effects
Alpha Lipoic acid information - learn about alpha lipoic acid benefits and ala side
www.bodybuildingforyou.com/health.../alpha-lipoic-acid.htm

Alpha Lipoic acid health benefits and nutritional information
Learn about alpha Lipoic acid, what its benefits and side effects are as well as how you can add it to your diet to improve your health.
www.alphalipoicacid.com

Dimethylaminoethanol

Dimethylethanolamine - Wikipedia, the free encyclopedia
Dimethylaminoethanol, also known as DMAE or dimethylethanolamine, is an organic compound.
en.wikipedia.org/wiki/Dimethylethanolamine

DMAE / Dimethylaminoethanol Supplements & Products
Buy DMAE supplements and products that contain DMAE.
www.herbalremedies.com/dmdidiamet.html

Shopping results for DMAE (dimethylaminoethanol)
Perricone MDDMAE(dimethyl amino ethanol) with Tocotrienols $30.00 new
Amazon.com

DMAE*(dimethylaminoethanol)* 100 Tablet
VitaminLife

DMAE - Health-Marketplace.com - Natural Health Products, Herbal ...
www.health-marketplace.com/DMAE.htm

DMAE *(Dimethylaminoethanol) Supplement Review*
Guide and Information about DMAE (*Dimethylaminoethanol*).
www.criticalbench.com/DMAE-Supplement-Review.htm

Oxygen Water Spray

Swiss O2 *Spray Oxygen Water Spray* Product Presentation
Just *spray* a misty breeze of SWISS O 2 SPRAY *on* your face and body and. Stimulating Boosting Vitalizing & Refreshing. Oxygenated Water – Use to .of SWISS O 2 *SPRAY* moisturizes and replenishes the *natural* elements of your skin allowing it to breathe.
www.slideshare.net/fleckenstein/swiss-o2-spray-product-presentation

Evian *natural spring water* - Shop sales, stores & prices at...
Tone, *refresh*, invigorate and moisturize *your* skin. Evian Mineral *Water Spray* ... below 7 is Acidic) ORP (*Oxygen* Reduction Potential) Best has negative value ... Evian Brumisateur *Facial Spray*.
www.thefind.com/food/browse-evian-natural-spring-water

Oxygenated Water Spray-Oxygenated Water Spray *Manufacturers*
Swiss O2 *Spray* is an *Oxygenated Water Spray* for instant *refreshment* of Skin & Body! Swiss O2 *Spray* is an all *natural* product! Contact now. Plus Liquid Oxygen Replenishing *Spring Water*
www.alibaba.com/showroom/oxygenated-water-spray.html

Evian Water Spray - Compare Prices, Reviews and Buy at NexTag .
Evian Spray Natural Mineral Water Facial Spray, 10.1 oz. Quantity No user ratings [rate this item] ... Tone refreshes, invigorate and moisturize *your* skin. .... So2s *Water Spray* 1.7oz *Oxygenated*
www.nextag.com/evian-water-spray/search-html

Botulinum toxin

Botulinum toxin - Wikipedia, the free encyclopedia
Botulinum toxin is a medication and a neurotoxin protein produced by the bacterium Clostridium Botulinum, and is known to be very toxic
en.wikipedia.org/wiki/Botulinum_toxin

Botulinum Toxin
Botulinum toxin has been used since 1980 to treat many muscle disorders such ...*Botulinum toxin* type A is specifically indicated for the lines between the ...
www.aad.org/public/publications/.../cosmetic_botulinum.html

How does Botox dissipate inside our body?
Doctor answers on Read 6 doctor answers to "How *does Botox* dissipate inside our body? ... Even if some molecules were to *go* into the bloodstream and travel to distant
www.realself.com

Dermal Fillers

Restylane® or Perlane®
Official Restylane® USA Website
www.RestylaneUSA.com

Dermal Fillers
Dermal Filler with Dermal Filler Treatment Call Jupiter's #1 Medical Spa
Jupiter Laser Medspa.com

Dermal Fillers - Restylane, Collagen and Radiance Information
Dermal fillers are used to reverse the effects of aging by reducing or eliminating wrinkles and replacing soft-tissue loss. Dermal fillers include collagen
www.dermanetwork.org/information/dermalfillers.asp

Dermal Fillers - Cosmetic *Dermal Filler* Q&A for Consumers
View answers to common questions about *dermal fillers* and the safety, risks, allergies, approved uses, age limit and products not approved by the FDA.
www.yourplasticsurgeryguide.com/...fillers/dermal-fillers-faq.htm

Dermal Fillers: eMedicine Dermatology by RS Bader
Overview: Perhaps nothing is more gratifying for cosmetic patients than having an immediate correction of rhytides or scars as a result
emedicine.medscape.com

Natural Fillers

POLYMER NANOCOMPOSITES: SYNTHETIC AND NATURAL
FILLERS. A REVIEW. William Gacitua E. 1 – Aldo Ballerini A.2 – Jinwen Zhang 3. ABSTRACT ...
www.scielo.cl/pdf/maderas/v7n3/art02.pdf

Botox Natural Fillers, Sculptra, Restylane, Perlane, Juvederm
Expert in Botox *Natural Fillers*, SCULPTRA®, Thermage, Carboxy therapy - LISA A. ZDINAK, MD
www.precisionaestheticsmd.com/services_botox_natural_fillers.html

HowStuffWorks "Natural Dermal Fillers"
Natural dermal *fillers* are also available.
Visit How Stuff Works to learn about *natural* dermal *fillers*.
health.howstuffworks.com

Collagen Injections

Molecular Therapy - Can Type VII Collagen Injections Cure
Remington et al. treated severely affected Col7a1 null mice with repeated intradermal *injections* of
recombinant full-length human *type* VII *collagen* (*type* ...
www.nature.com

COLLAGEN - Why Anti aging Skincare *Collagen*?
Botox *Injection* you don't need surgery or *collagen* replacement therapy for .Our protein is
type I *collagen*. When consumed *collagen* in Colvita is only
www.collagenelife.com

Collagen injection*s* for beauty enhancement
Human collagen is a bioengineered product and comes from a human donor. This *type* of collagen
injection usually does not require any kind of skin test ...
www.plasticsurgeryadvisor.com/.../collagen-injections.

Injection of recombinant human *type* VII collagen
Injection of recombinant human *type* VII *collagen* restores *collagen* function in dystrophic
epidermolysis bullosa. Woodley DT, Keene DR, Atha T, Huang Y
www.ncbi.nlm.nih.gov/pubmed/15195089

Collagen - Wikipedia, the free encyclopedia
With *type* I *collagen* and possibly all fibrillar *collagens* if not all. Over 90% of the *collagen* in the
body, however, is of *type* I, II, III, and IV.
en.wikipedia.org/wiki/Collagen

Collagen Injections
Give it to me straight...What happens during *Collagen* Filler *injections*? Allergy test. Depending on
the *type* of *collagen* you and your plastic surgeon choose ...
www.plasticsurgery.org/Patients_and.../Collagen_Fillers.

Autologen

Injectable Dermal Filler - Autologous human collagen (*Autologen*)
Skin care and rejuvenation information and reviews based on published research and other
independent sources. Injectable Dermal Filler - Autologous
www.smartskincare.com

Autologen | Information and tips on *Autologen*
Autologen is a newer form of collagen injections. Unlike Collagen (derived from cows and
trademarked) and Dermalogen (collagen derived from human tissue ...
www.beauty-cosmetic-guide.com/beauty/autologen.htm

Self-Derivative Injectable Products
Autologen: (technically: Autologous human collagen) this injectable collagen is derived from the
patient's own skin which is removed at
www.yestheyrefake.net/injectable_fillers_selfderived.htm

Injectable Fillers

RU (Russia) Injectable Fillers - Plastic Surgery Portal
Collagen should be injected into your skin only by a trained health care professional. By supplementing your skin`s own *collagen*, Dermalogen is collagen extracted from deceased
immersivemedical.com/injectable-fillers_ru_2

Malaysia (MY) *Injectable Fillers* - Plastic Surgery Portal
Collagen should be injected into your skin only by a trained health care professional. By supplementing your skin`s own *collagen*, ... Dermalogen is collagen extracted from deceased human donors. It`s also called injectable Human Tissue Matrix.
immersivemedical.com/injectable-fillers Malaysia

Hylaform

Hylaform.Ca - Hyaluronic Acid Dermal Filler
Mar 18, 2005 ... *Hylaform* is an injectable wrinkle filler to be used for the treatment of moderate to severe facial wrinkles and folds.
www.hylaform.ca

Hylaform - Treatment & Injection Information
Hylaform is hyaluronic acid dermal filler used for wrinkle treatment. Hylaform *is* injected into the dermis to replenish dermal volume loss
www.dermanetwork.org/information/hylaform.asp

Hylaform - Instant wrinkle filler in Orange County, California
Hylaform, Captique, Restylane, Cosmoderm and Cosmoplast are used to remove wrinkles, augment and plump lips and correct facial
www.totaldermatology.com/pages/hylaform.html

SIDE EFFECTS OF HYLAFORM
As with any medical treatment, there are side effects of *HylaForm* that patients should understand before seeking this treatment. *Hylaform* is a non-invasive ...
www.aboardcertifiedplasticsurgeonresource.com/hylaform/side-

Stem Cells

Stem cell - Wikipedia, the free encyclopedia
Stem cells are cells found in all multi cellular organisms. They are characterized by the ability to renew themselves through mitotic cell division and
en.wikipedia.org/wiki/Stem cell

Stem Cell Basics [*Stem Cell* Information]
Apr 28, 2009 ... Primer providing basic information about *stems cells*.
stemcells.nih.gov/info/basics

NIH Stem Cell Information Home Page
Apr 29, 2010 ... Official resource about research, using human embryonic lines under Federal policy, eligibility criteria, funding opportunities for
stemcells.nih.gov

Laser Skin Resurfacing

Laser Skin Resurfacing - Skin Procedure Growing in Popularity

Apr 12, 2010 ... What's more, today's lasers are gentler and safer than they have been in the past. .Which is more invasive and far less gentle than microdermabrasion in 2008, 103394 of the laser skin resurfacing techniques performed have undergone laser skin
www.yourplasticsurgeryguide.com/laser-skin.../laser-skin-resurfacing

Skin Rejuvenation Treatment| Atlanta Laser Clinic

Microdermabrasion is a procedure that uses fine crystals and a controlled vacuum to exfoliate the skin. ... Chemical Peels are a category of advanced clinical skin rejuvenation ...Dermabrasion is a procedure in which a medical professional
www.atlantalaserclinic.com/skinrejuvenation.html

Benefits of Laser Skin Rejuvenation with Cool Touch Technology

The Vita-K Chemical Peel is one of the latest skin rejuvenation treatments consider the key benefits of laser and light therapy for skin rejuvenation. ... For aging skin; it is a variation of the Intense Pulsed Light procedure, as laser skin a series of chemical
www.locateadoc.com

Skin Rejuvenation Articles

The Sciton Micro Laser Peel is one of the latest innovative treatments available for ... for aging skin; it is a variation of the Intense Pulsed Light procedure, the key benefits of laser and light therapy for skin rejuvenation. Thinking about microdermabrasion?
www.locateadoc.com/articles/skin-rejuvenation

Spa Treatment

Spa Treatment - What Is A Spa Treatment?

What is a *spa treatment*?
Here's an introduction to *spa treatments*, including massage, facials and body treatments.
spas.about.com/cs/spatreatments/a/treatmentchioce.htm

Spas - Spa Treatments

A look at the spa menu can be overwhelming. Should I get a massage or body treatment? Hydrate or detoxify? Find more about what *spa treatments*.
spas.about.com/od/massage/Spa_Treatments.htm

Collagen Induction Therapy

Collagen Induction Therapy

Apr 15, 2010 ... The *Collagen-Induction-Therapy* (*CIT*) by micro-needling the skin requires special medical ... This body reaction is called neo-*collagenesis*. ...
www.dermaroller.de/en/medical-dermaroller

Canberra's Day Spa - Collagen Induction Therapy (*CIT*)

(Neo-*collagenesis*) as well as in new capillaries for an improved blood supply (neo-angiogenis). This procedure is called *Collagen Induction Therapy* (*CIT* ...
www.ginashumantuning.com.au/Pages2008/CIT.htm

Dr. Philip Miller New York City Plastic Surgery: Wrinkles and...

Collagen Channeling for Natural *Collagen Induction Therapy*: ... the more collagen can be made. Therefore, allowing natural *collagenesis* to occur. Find More Information on Roll-*Cit* which helps reduce wrinkles and acne scars. ...
www.drphilipmiller.com

Medical ROLL-*CIT*

MEDICAL ROLL-*CIT*™, Collagen Channeling for Natural *Collagen Induction Therapy*. Many clinicians believe that laser resurfacing is the most ...
www.environ.co.za/contents/.../roll_cit/roll_cit_medical.htm

Environ Roll *Cit* | Focus *Cit* | Ionzyme DF Machine | Environ Skincare

Collagen Channeling for Natural *Collagen Induction Therapy*. The Environ® Cosmetic Roll-*Cit*™ is the latest revolutionary design from Environ® in skin care ...
environ-skin-care.com/environ-roll-cit/

Laser Treatments

Does laser skin treatment stimulate collagen production*?*

Laser treatments do stimulate the production of collagen in the dermal layer of the skin. ... *It is* actually the thermal *(*heat*)* injury induced by the lasers which ... *I* prefer to use fractional CO2 lasers as they combine safety and efficacy.
www.realself.com

Sublative rejuvenation: experience with a new fractional

Unlike *fractional* ablative *laser treatments*, which can disrupt 10-70% of the epidermis ...creating controlled *thermal* damage in the *dermis stimulates* a wound healing wound .after and between all the treatments to enhance *collagen*
www.thefreelibrary.com

Gizmo's

Cool Health Gadgets *Gizmos* | Fitness Gadgets

June 21st, 2010 by Fit *Gizmos* Leave Your Comment Here! It's a high-end product that offers programs for general wellness, *anti-aging*, and play. ...
www.fitgizmos.com

Beauty Gadgets

Latest beauty gadgets and gizmos

Galvanic facial massager .Tags: anti-age cosmetics, anti-aging, beauty pills, dermasilk anti-wrinkle ...
www.fitgizmos.com/health/beautygadgets

Oh no! Another gizmo. Oxylift. Anyone tried it?

Oxylift, I got it at the international *anti*
 show... we got it for $100 a piece because there were 5 of us. I also saw it on sale at ...
www.essentialdayspa.com

Six Pack Abs Gizmo*s* Exercise - As Seen On TV

Derma logy *Anti Aging* Solution Revitol Hair Removal Cream ... A: For the $100 or so that this *gizmo* costs, there are better things you can
www.naturalherbalz.com/articles/six-packs-abs

Beauty Gizmo Review: Baby Quasar, Week 1 « The Gloss

Oct 24, 2007 ... Now, it's time for Beauty *Gizmo* to review, and give the real scoop. Primarily the routine would be for *anti-aging* – start
thegloss.com/articles/beauty-gizmo-review-baby-quasar-week-1-359/

Face Trainer

The FaceTrainer by no!no!
The no!no! Family does it again with the *FaceTrainer*™. The only device of its kind to be registered and listed with the FDA, the *FaceTrainer*™ combines ...
www.my-no-no.com/facetrainer_about.asp

Top 5 weirdest beauty buys: #1 the Face Trainer
The Face Trainer from no!no! You can lift weights to tone arms, hit the treadmill to tighten legs, and crunch your way to six-pack abs.
www.examiner.com/x-9539-NY-Beauty-Industry-

Face Trainer | The Frisky
Jun 10, 2009 ... Introducing "The *Face Trainer*," is a mask-helmet that you put over your whole head which creates resistance so when you move your facial.
www.thefrisky.com/tag/face+trainer

Growth Hormone

Growth hormone *treatment - Wikipedia, the free encyclopedia*
Growth hormone (*GH*) is a peptide hormone secreted by the pituitary gland that stimulates growth and cell reproduction. In the past growth hormone was ...
en.wikipedia.org/wik i/Growth_hormone_treatment

Growth Hormone
Aug 14, 2008 ... A *growth hormone* (*GH*) test measures the amount of human *growth hormone* (*GH*) in the blood. GH is made by the pituitary gland and is needed
www.webmd.com/a-to-z-guides/growth-hormone

Human *Growth Hormone*
Growth Hormone (*GH*) is the master hormone, because the master gland, the anterior pituitary gland, releases it. While GH is not necessary or critical to ...
gordonresearch.com

Hormone Replacement

Hormone Replacement Therapy
Aug 7, 2003 ... Description: *Hormone Therapy* (*HT*) or *Hormone Replacement Therapy* (*HRT*) is the giving of the female hormones estrogen and progesterone,
www.healthinsite.gov.au/.

Menopause - information, symptoms and treatments
Hormone replacement therapy (*HRT*) replaces some of the hormones that are reduced. Health care guideline: menopause and *hormone therapy* (*HT*): collaborative. Association and the Royal Pharmaceutical Society of Great *Britain*, 2009 ...
hcd2.bupa.co.uk

Biodentiacals

Are *Biodenticals* for you? Hormonal Contraceptive
Dec 19, 2006 ... There are many ways women may choose to manage their hormonal health after a hysterectomy, the birth of a child or even just as a supplement ...
www.syl.com

Suzanne Somers staves off Menopause with Biodenticals - Monsters...
Feb 1, 2009 ... Actress Suzanne Somers promotes a natural real food diet, and says if you pick it, pluck it, shoot it or milk it is okay to ingest.
www.monstersandcritics.com/

Biodenticals hormone pellet under the skin.
These pellets are identical to the hormones. I am due soon for my second round of the Biodentical treatment ...
www.innerrealm.net/biodenticals.html

First Suzanne Somers, Next Oprah Winfrey Body Logic MD's
For the first time I feel there is hope after reading all about *Biodenticals* and Hormone imbalance. Between the brain fog, hot flashes,
bodylogicmd.wordpress.com

IV Drip Vitamin Cocktails

IV Drip Vitamin Cocktails*: Latest Anti-Aging Secret or 'Quackery ...*
Feb 8, 2010 ... Move over, Botox. You're not the only needle in town. Popular in Japan for the past year and now gaining appeal in the USA, *IV drip vitamin* ...
www.stylelist.com/

Institute for Healing Arts
Myers' *Cocktail*, an *intravenous vitamin* nutrient supplement, was formulated more than 30 years ago by John Myers, MD, a Baltimore physician. ...
www.healingartsresearch.org/B-2-b-IV-Vit.htm

Canadians turning to *"vitamin cocktails"* to boost energy, health
Mar 12, 2010 ... She heard about these so-called "*vitamin cocktails*" through friends ...Another vitamin *intravenous* gaining popularity is one that includes ...
www.vancouversun.com/health/...vitamin+cocktails.../story.htm

Chelation IV Therapy

Chelation IV Therapy
SunridgeMedical.com/Cancer Care .Safe Effective Chelation IV Cancer Therapy. To Learn More start Here."EDTA Chelation Warning"
www.improvedoralchelation.com/

Looking for Chelation?
www.CardioRenew.com

Full Explanation Of *Intravenous Chelation Therapy* -- IV Chelation
This is the best description of intravenous chelation therapy on the Internet
www.oralchelation.com/technical/IV1.html

The World Of *Intravenous Chelation Therapy* Is Crumbling!
May 20, 2008.Now, let's look at a series of two *intravenous chelation therapy* sessions. These are normally about 3 hours each, so these two sessions ...
www.oralchelation.com/LifeGlowBasic/description/p10.htm

I.V. Chelation Therapy
How does *chelation therapy* work? For most of these metals, an intravenous solution of vitamins, minerals, and the chelator EDTA is prepared. ...
www.anti-agingmd.com/chelation.html

Demi Moore - Leech Therapy

Demi Moore Twitters With Dave *Letterman*, Sits In His Lap (VIDEO)
Apr 21, 2010 ... *Demi Moore* joined *David Letterman* Monday night, and he looked thrilled when she got up from her seat to come around and sit on his lap. ...
www.huffingtonpost.com/.../demi-moore-twitters-with_n_545835

Demi Moore visits "Late Show With *David Letterman*" | www...
Apr 20, 2010 *Demi Moore* visits "Late Show With *David Letterman*" at the Ed Sullivan Theater on April 20, 2010 in New York City. ...
bricksandstonesgossip.com/

Demi Moore*:* "Late Show With *David Letterman*" Video: Top Socialite
Mar 25, 2008. Demi Moore (she's 45 by the way! holy crap!) stopped by David Letterman's
www.topsocialite.com

Skull-lift

Give me a *skull-lift* - Times Online
Nov 17, 2007 ... Scientists have found that sagging skin is not itself to blame for making us look older – it's our sagging *skulls*.
women.timesonline.co.uk/tol/life_and./article2882846.ece

Facing the future - Telegraph
How about a *skull-lift*? Or a fat-harvested bust augmentation? From stem-cell injections to *skull-lifts*, the industry is on the cusp of
www.telegraph.co.uk/fashion

Face Lifts are So Last Century. Try a Skull Lift I instead. | Jewcy.com
Jan 23, 2008 ... Subhead (DEK): Have we learned nothing from Jocelyn Wildenstein? Body: The Bride of Wildenstein: a cautionary tale. The Bride of Wildenstein: a ...
www.jewcy.com

Non Surgical Face-Lifts

Non Surgical Face Lifts - Do They Work?
Red & Blue LED Light Therapy for Face & Neck. *Anti-Aging* Phototherapy.... I've heard of the fat-dissolving machines but the only ones I've *come* across use ultrasound, *not* red light.... *Yes*, I had noticed our Hub Pages experience is very
www.hubpages.com/hub/nonsurgical-facelift

Awful Plastic Surgery: Ten Worst Celebrity Facelifts!
Dedicated to exploring the *next generation* of Body and Mind Enhancement.
The worst part of his plastic *surgery* is his too tight face *lift*. 'Rocky' Dennis (played by Eric Stoltz) a boy with a massive *skull* deformity. How much would *you* pay for
www.body-philosophy.net/Awful_Plastic_Surgery_Celebrity

Sagging Cheeks Lift Using Facial Exercise
There was a time that *anti-aging* options were limited to mostly skin care lotions. Remember, you may not see complications immediately but they can rear their ugly. Over the *next* seven weeks *you* will teach yourself the simple yet easy steps to Plastic
www.articlesbase.com

Cosmetic Surgery

Cosmetic Surgery Procedures | Before and After Photos | Find...
CosmeticSurgery.com is an educational online resource providing a wide range of information related to *cosmetic surgery* procedures.
www.cosmeticsurgery.com

Cosmetic Plastic *Surgery* Consumer Guide - Find a Plastic Surgeon
Consumer Guide to Plastic *Surgery* is the top online resource for information about plastic *surgery* and *cosmetic* enhancements, and how to choose a surgeon.
www.yourplasticsurgeryguide.com

American Academy of *Cosmetic Surgery* (AACS) - Welcome
Not-for-profit organization providing information on *cosmetic surgery* for patients, physicians, and the media, includes a physician search and procedural.
www.cosmeticsurgery.org

Face-lift (Rhytidectomy)

Facelift *(Rhytidectomy)* Cosmetic Surgery Procedure Information
If you are bothered by the signs of aging *in your* face, *a* facelift *may* ... *a* surgical procedure *to improve* visible signs of aging in the face *and neck, such as:* ....Rhytidectomy*: A* surgical procedure *also known as* facelift,
www.plasticsurgery.org/.../Procedures/...Procedures/Facelift.html

Facelift / Face Lift *(Rhytidectomy)* — Risks, Benefits
A *face lift*, or *Rhytidectomy*, is a *surgical procedure* used to *reduce facial* ... your *facial* contour, it can also cause nerve damage, *visible* scarring, swelling, Men are now turning to *Rhytidectomy* to
www.docshop.com

Consumers - Procedures - Head - Facelift | The American Society
The *face* usually portrays the first *visible signs of aging*. This information will be used to formulate a *surgical* plan and the goals of the *procedure* will: The *facelift procedure* usually involves incisions in front of and behind the ear, Avoidance of factors that could
www.surgery.org/consumers/procedures/head/facelift

Face lift *(Rhytidectomy)* - skin care cosmetic treatments
Face lift surgery is a cosmetic *procedure* that involves redirecting ... as the term *Rhytidectomy* (which literally means "*surgical* ... After the surgery, a pressure bandage will be applied to the *face* to *reduce* the risk of hematoma for their ability to
skin-care.health-cares.net/face-lift.php

Number of procedures in the USA
http://www.answers.com/topic/plastic-surgery

Rhytidectomy

Face Lifts: Before and After Photos *Face Lift* **Pictures**
Before and after pictures of *Face* Lifts, (*Rhytidectomy* Surgery).
Information on *face-lift* surgery (*Rhytidectomy*) including average costs,
www.smartplasticsurgery.com/facelifts_ba.html

Facelift *(Rhytidectomy)* **Cosmetic Surgery Procedure Information**
If you are bothered by the *signs of aging* in your *face*, a *facelift* may be a *surgical procedure* to
improve *visible signs of aging in the face* and neck, such as: *Rhytidectomy*: *surgical procedure* also
www.plasticsurgery.org/Patients_and.../Facelift.html

Face Lift Surgery (*Rhytidectomy***) Pictures - Before & After Photos**
Video Insight. View your *procedure* in 3D. Common Questions & Answers about *Face Lift* Surgery
(*Rhytidectomy*) ... Non *Surgical* Rhinoplasty, Non-*Surgical* Cosmetic Procedures.... California was
unhappy with her facial *aging* changes. .
www.locateadoc.com/.../face-lift-surgery-rhytidectomy.html

Facelift - Guide to Face Lift Surgery - Risks, Cost & Benefits
Find the best *face lift* variation for you. View before & after photos and ... on the *facelift procedure*,
what makes a good *facelift* surgery candidate: *Facelift* cosmetic surgery (*Rhytidectomy*) is intended
to improve your ... than a *facelift*, using radio waves to
www.yourplasticsurgeryguide.com/face-lift

Sheila Jeffrey's

Sheila Jeffrey's **- SSPS**
Faculty of Arts School of *Social and Political Sciences*. Links: University Homepage, about
the Assoc. *Prof. Sheila Jeffrey's. Prof. Sheila Jeffrey's*. I am originally from the UK and came to
the *University of Melbourne* in 1991.Not for Sale, Melbourne, *Australia*:
www.ssps.unimelb.edu.au

The School of *Social and Political Sciences*
Offers a wide range of courses and ... *Prof.* Robyn Eckersley - The Future of Carbon Trading
www.ssps.unimelb.edu.au

Sheila Jeffreys **- Wikipedia, the free encyclopedia**
She is a *professor* in *Political Science* at the *University of Melbourne* in *Australia,* These concepts
made to fit changing *social* conditions: the New Woman was. in the United Kingdom:
en.wikipedia.org

Associate *Professor Sheila Jeffrey's* **PhD**
School of *Social and Political Sciences. University of Melbourne.*
University of Western *Australia* Press. J *effreys, Sheila* 2000:
plataforma8demarzo.org/.../CV_corto%20_Sheila_Jeffreys.pdf

PROF SHEILA JEFFREYS
PROF *SHEILA JEFFREYS* (*Social and Political Sciences*) Female-to-male... Find an Expert
Profiling the *University of Melbourne's* Researchers Judicial child abuse: The family court
www.findanexpert.unimelb.edu.au/.../person14541.html

The Ugly Side of Beauty

Channel 4 - TV Listings - Tuesday 3rd of August 2010
The *Ugly* Face of *Beauty*. *Dr Christian Jessen* hosts this ultimate guide to
New series. Experts with diametrically opposed approaches put their ...
www.channel4.com/tv-listings/daily/2010/08/03

The Atkins Diet: Fat or Fiction - Channel 4
This documentary explores al *sides* of the popular - and so-called 'miracle' - diet. ... *Ugly* Face
of *Beauty* · Supersize vs Super skinny Dr Christian Jessen ...
www.channel4.

UK TV *Documentary* shows UK TV listings - ITV1 Granada
Channel 4 Today 08:00pm, The Ugly Face of Beauty *(Documentary)*, Series examining the
booming cosmetic surgery industry with *Dr Christian Jessen*. ...
tvchitchat.co.uk/genre/Documentary -

Seroma

Seroma - Wikipedia, the free encyclopedia
A seroma *is a* pocket of clear serous fluid that sometimes develops in the body after surgery. When
small blood vessels are ruptured, blood plasma can seep ...
en.wikipedia.org/wiki/Seroma

Mastectomy and *Seroma* - OrganizedWisdom Health
Jun 10, 2010 A *seroma* is a *pocket of clear serous fluid that sometimes develops in the body after
surgery*. ... When *small blood vessels are ruptured, blood plasma can* seep out; inflammation
caused by dying injured cells
organizedwisdom.com

Chapter 11

Final Words

Healthy diet
en.wikipedia.org/wiki/Healthydiet

Food standards agency UK – Healthy diet
www.eatwell.gov.uk/healthydiet/

5 A DAY - Live Well - NHS Choices
Introduction to *5 A DAY* portions of fruit and vegetables, including portion size,
www.5aday.nhs.uk

Quorn

Quorn -They're versatile and quick to cook - but what are they made of?
Find out how we make Quorn foods and what makes them so good for you
www.quorn.co.uk

Marlow Foods Ltd
Have put time and effort into coming up with the perfect solution. The Quorn™ range consists of a
selection of versatile products which
ww.quorn.com

Quorn - Wikipedia, the free encyclopedia
As a result, Marlow Foods decided to sell *Quorn* as a healthy meat alternative *Quorn* is the leading brand in the UK's £582 million *vegetarian* market
en.wikipedia.org/wiki/Quorn

Protein Powder& Vitamins

What is Protein Powder?
18 Jul 2010 ... *Protein powder* is designed to be taken every day as a dietary *supplement*. Even if you aren't a bodybuilder, starting your day with a *protein* ...
wwwwi.segeek.com/what-is-protein-powder.htm

Whey Protein Powder Benefits - Whey Protein Information
Whey *protein powder* benefits and whey *protein supplement* information and whey *protein... Vitamin* K *Supplements* .Popular Diet *Pills* & Fat Burners ... The differences in the
www.bodybuildingforyou.com

How Vitamins *Work – Working* For Us | HowItWorks.net
25 Aug 2008 ... So we know *vitamins* are vital, now let's meet them individually, find out some of the places where *they* can be found, and what *they do*. ...
www.howitworks

Vitamins what *they* are and how *they work*
Vitamins: *Vitamins* what *they* are and how *they work*. A vitamin is an organic molecule whose insufficiency in the diet can result in disease. ...
www.health-garden.com/vitamins/index

Vitamin tablets 'may *do* more harm than good' | Mail Online
Vitamin supplements *do* not *work* and may *do* more harm than good while *vitamins* may ward off disease in the test-tube; *they do* little to ...
www.dailymail.co.uk/health/article

Vitamins and Supplements: *Do They Work*? - US News and World
9 Dec 2008 ... The picture is mixed, but thumbs up for vitamin D and fish oil.
health.usnews.com

TTC - Any good vitamins/ do they work? - Yahoo! UK & Ireland Answers
Hiya Girlies I have been TTC for 7 cycles now and getting desperate: Dandy dear, good for you to be proactive in finding ways to be more effective in ...
uk.answers.yahoo.com

Metabolism

Metabolism - Wikipedia, the free encyclopedia
Metabolism is the set of chemical reactions that happen in living organisms to maintain life. These processes allow organisms to grow and reproduce,
en.wikipedia.org/wiki/Metabolism

Metabolism
The human body gets energy from food through *metabolism*. Brush up on *metabolism* basics in this
kidshealth.org

Dieting and Metabolism
How dieting affects metabolism and how to increase metabolic rate
www.weightlossresources.co.uk/calories/.../starvation.htm

Soft Drinks

Soft drink - Wikipedia, the free encyclopedia
A soft drink (also referred to as soda, pop, soda pop, coke or *fizzy drink*) is a drink that typically contains no alcohol, though may contain small amounts...
en.wikipedia.org/wiki/Soft drink

Minciu Sodas - Global Teams of Independent Thinkers
Contact Andrius Kulikauskas, Direktorius of Minciu Sodas, ms@ms.lt, +370 699 30003, skype: minciusodas or visit our chat room or leave a note at any of our
www.ms.lt/

How Much Sugar in Sodas and Beverages?
Everyone knows that soda is packed with sugar. We stacked up the sugar in some average sized bottles, plus 7-Eleven's super-sized line of Gulp beverages. ...
www.sugarstacks.com/beverages.htm

Energy drink - Wikipedia, the free encyclopedia
Energy drinks are soft drinks advertised as boosting energy. These drinks usually do not emphasize energy derived from the calories they
en.wikipedia.org

Salt

Salt - Wikipedia, the free encyclopedia
Salt is a mineral that is composed primarily of sodium chloride. It is essential for animal life in small quantities, but is harmful to animals and plants ...
en.wikipedia.org/wiki/Salt

Food Standards Agency - Eat well, be well - *Salt*
Are you having too much *salt*? You might not think so. But every day 26 million adults in the UK eat too much *salt*. You could be eating too
www.eatwell.gov.uk/healthydiet/fss/salt

So Natural Gourmet Salt
Himalayan Pink salt from £3.50; Black Lava, Oak Smoked; Red Alaea
www.himalayancrystalsalt.co.uk

Himalayan Crystal Salt
www.amazinghealth.co.uk

Natural Salt, Purest in the World With over 78 minerals
Himalayan Crystal Salt contains over 80 essential minerals and trace elements. Buy and learn more about the power of salt.
www.himalayancrystalsalt.co.uk

Original Himalayan Crystal Salt
The One, The Only, The Original *Himalayan Crystal Salt*.
www.himalayancrystalsalt.com

Professor Stuart Warden

Phys Ed: Does Ibuprofen Help or Hurt During Exercise? - Well Blog...
1 Sep 2009....has become a ritual," says Stuart Warden, *an assistant* professor *and* director of physical therapy research at Indiana University,
well.blogs.nytimes.com/2009

285

Collagen: House of Verona
Professor Stuart Warden, Director of Physical Therapy Research at Indiana University, informed the New York Times last week that "the stresses of exercise activate a particular molecular pathway that increases collagen," which leads to
bookings@houseofverona.com

Dr. Stuart Warden, PhD, PT, FACSM: *Physical Therapy*: School of
Department of Physical Therapy: IU School of Health & Rehabilitation Sciences .Assistant Professor *and* Director *of* Research, Department of *Physical Therapy*, Journal of Orthopedic and shrs.iupui.edu/about/profile.php?emp

Exercise Increases Collagen;
11 Sep 2009 ... Professor Stuart Warden, Director of Physical Therapy Research at Indiana University, informed the New York Times last week that "the stresses of exercise activate a particular molecular pathway that increases collagen," which
houseofverona.com/exercise-increases-collagen-ibuprofen-inhibits

Dr. Oz

Facial Exercises: A New Wrinkle | Beauty Bunch
30 Apr 2010... What *Oz* wrote in the book, he mentioned on his show *a* Japanese study that may give credence to the idea that facial exercises work. ...
www.beautybunch.com/2010/04/30/facial-exercises

Facial Exercises: A New Wrinkle | Beauty Bunch
30 Apr 2010 ... Although *Dr. Oz* didn't originally endorse facial exercises in his '08 ... and safe for their faces, especially since facial exercise works! ...
www.beautybunch.com/

Dr Perricone

Skin Firming Tips for Better Skin
24 Nov 2009. Simple facial exercises are great for tightening the skin of the face. For the rest of your body, it is great to engage in simple
blog.perriconemd.com/skin-firming-tips-for-better-skin

April 2010 Newsletter
On his Blog Page, MD Perricone, he *states that, "If your skin has already begun to lose its tone and elasticity, natural face* lift options are available. ...
www.facercise.com

Dr. Berman

Learn about Mark Berman MD, FACS
Dr. *Berman's* full Curriculum Vitae with Hospital Affiliations, Societies and Media Appearances.
www.markbermanmd.com/about.aspx

Dr. Berman - Cosmetic Surgeon
Mark Berman, M.D., F.A.C.S... Cosmetic surgeon since 1551 Ocean Avenue, suite 200. Santa Monica, CA 90401. Phone: 310-394-0570. Fax: 310-394-6710 ...
www.westland.net/berman

Dr. Mark Berman, MD, of Los Angeles, Named President of the...
4 Mar 2010 Dr. *Mark Berman*, *MD*, of Los Angeles, has been named President of the American
Academy of Cosmetic Surgery for 2010. Berman's appointment was
www.plasticsurgeonsnews.com

Mark Berman, M.D., *F.A.C.S.*
20 Feb 2009 ... *Mark Berman*, *M.D.*, F.A.C.S... Dr. Berman discusses breast augmentation. Santa
Monica plastic surgeon talks about the latest develop
wellnesshour.com
Dr Margaret Olsen

Dr. Margaret E Olsen Kohner, MD - Dermatology - *Los Angeles, CA*
Dermatology, Check Doctor reports, ratings, credentials, information, background, complaints
www.healthgrades.com

Margaret Olsen, MD *Dermatologist in* Los Angeles, CA *90025*
Margaret Olsen, MD is a Dermatologist at 11600 Wilshire Blvd Ste 406 *Los Angeles, CA.*
Wellness.com provides reviews, contact information, driving
www.wellness.com

MEDICAL ENDORSEMENTS - Discover youthful beauty with
Past President of the *California* Academy of Cosmetic Surgeons ... Carolyn Doherty, *M.D*... Beverly
Hills, *CA* ... *Margaret Olsen, M.D*... Los Angeles, *CA* ...
www.cynthiarowland.com/medical_endorse.php

Cynthia Rowland Successful Aging Expert, Author and Motivational
She has been interviewed by many publications, including The *Los Angeles* Times, The New York
Daily News and The ... "Margaret Olsen, M.D. Los Angeles, CA ...
www.selfgrowth.com

Chinese Facial Exercises

Chinese facial exercises & massage techniques invigorate your face
Traditional Chinese facial exercises include acupressure, massage & stretching to relax & tone
facial muscles, improve local blood flow & relieve problems ...
www.chinese-holistic-health-exercises.com/facial-exercises.html

TIDP REPORT
Visit to Dong Jiao Min Xiang Primary School in Beijing, *China*. ... Everyday the whole *school*
exercises in the playground to a type of drill and then to ... day music is piped into the classroom
and the children work on facial exercises. ...
www.lgfl.net/lgfl/leas

Do Chinese *Facial Exercises* | LIVESTRONG.COM
18 Nov 2009 ... Diet & Nutrition · Diet & Nutrition for *Children* ... To do Chinese *facial exercises*, you
must learn the location of the ... In *China*, many believe wrinkles indicate a stagnant life force
energy, which they call Chi.
www.livestrong.com/article/6626-do-chinese-facial-exercises

Eye Exercises to Improve Learning and Visual Attention
Eye Exercises for Better Visual Health... Focus when looking from near to far, such as when
children have to look from their desks to the board at *school*. .... These ancient Chinese puzzles
work much like electronic parquetry blocks. ...
www.eyecanlearn.com

Eye Exercises Blog
Permalink -- click for full blog post *"Chinese Eye Exercises"* ... Permalink -- click for full blog post "The Prevention Of Myopia In School Children" ...
www.eye-exercises-for-good-vision.com/eye-exercises-blog.html

Eye Exercises for Myopia
The Chinese eye exercises are based on acupressure points and have been practiced ... the *eye exercises* for myopia? Prevention of Myopia in *School Children* ...
www.eye-exercises-for-good-vision.com

Videos for China school children eye exercises Chinese Eye Exercises
www.youtube.com

Instant Facelift Transforms Your Face Without Cosmetic Surgery
7 Jun 2010 ... *Facial exercise* works better than electrical toning and has been practiced in *China* regularly for thousands of years. ...
www.healthynewage.com/facelift.html

Facial Muscle *Exercises* Bring an Appearance of Youth – NTDTV.com
23 Jun 2010 ... But how many people know about the benefits of *facial exercises*? In the meeting of "La nobel estetics", certified Cosmetician Ilana Keren ...
english.ntdtv.com

Anti-aging | Health Articles | *Facial Exercise* Techniques
To choose which *facial exercise* program best suits your facelift without surgery ... United States, India, *China*, Costa Rica, England, Malaysia, Singapore, ...
www.worldwidehealth.com

Facial Paralysis, Bell's Palsy, surgery information, FAQ, causes
Chinese *face* reading is an ancient art that has been developed over centuries, not only in *China* but over the wider area of Asia owing to *China's* cultural ...
www.facialparalysisinstitute.com

ORIENTAL MEDICAL CENTER: SERVICES - CHINESE FACIAL THERAPY
Chinese *Facial* Therapy uses ancient *Chinese* theory in combination with modern *facial* techniques to provide our patients with an effective way to look and ...
www.orientalmedicalcenter.com/services_facial.html

Contact

Visit us
Email
Guestbook
Customer Service
Where to buy Fitface
www.Fitfacetoning.com

Follow on Twitter
www.twitter.com/Fitfacetoning

Read our blog
www.blog .Fitfacetoning.com

Watch us on YouTube
www.youtube.com/user/Fitfacetoning
Fitface fun exercises
See Charlotte on ABC News at 5pm WPBF
Fitface professional instructor training
Fitface seminar

Coupon

Free **entrance** to any seminar worldwide held by
Charlotte Hamilton

Or

Free introductory **lesson** offered by
Fitface hands free toning

Or

Free, next/revised, **publication**
of
Fitface hands free toning
printed or eBook

For further information
www.fitfacetoning.com